Placenta as a Model
and a Source

Placenta as a Model and a Source

Edited by
Olga Genbačev
INEP, Institute of Endocrinology, Immunology, and Nutrition
Zemun, Yugoslavia
Arnold Klopper
Department of Obstetrics and Gynaecology, University of Aberdeen
Aberdeen, Scotland, United Kingdom
and
Rebecca Beaconsfield
SCIP Research Unit, University of London
London, United Kingdom

Plenum Press • New York and London

Library of Congress Cataloging in Publication Data

Placenta as a model and a source / edited by Olga Genbačev, Arnold Klopper, and
  Rebecca Beaconsfield.
    p.   cm.
Based on a workshop held May 19–20, 1988, at INEP, Zemun, Yugoslavia.
Bibliography: p.
Includes index.

ISBN-13: 978-1-4612-8100-9   e-ISBN-13: 978-1-4613-0823-2
DOI: 10.1007/978-1-46113-0823-2

  1. Placenta—Physiology—Congresses. 2. Placenta—Cultures and culture media—
Congresses. 3. Placenta hormones—Congresses. I. Genbacev, Olga. II. Klopper, Arnold. III. Beaconsfield, Rebecca.
QP281.P542   1989   89-16113
612.6′3—dc20   CIP

Based, in part, on a workshop on Placenta as a Model and a Source,
held May 19–20, 1988, at INEP, Zemun, Yugoslavia

© 1989 Plenum Press, New York
Softcover reprint of the hardcover 1st edition 1989

A Division of Plenum Publishing Corporation
233 Spring Street, New York, N.Y. 10013

FOREWORD

The foreword to the "book of a meeting" is often an excuse for a paen of praise, a homily, or even an apologia - and sometimes a combination of all three. While certain traditions have been dispensed with in this volume the standard pattern for the foreword has its advantages, so here at least tradition will be adhered to - though in reverse order from that stated above.

The apologia can be dismissed briefly, for the editors have explained in their General Introduction that this is not the book of a meeting. All that remains to be added here is a description of the modus operandi. Being aware that speaking and writing are different activities requiring different presentation, each participant was asked to prepare a script for publication resembling what he would speak about only in outline. It may be that as a result the essays lack detail and are thin under some of the classical headings of scientific writing. So the reader, in turn, is asked to accept this and give his attention instead to the concepts and ideas contained therein. It may even come about that this kind of presentation will in the end result in something less ephemeral than the standard conference proceedings book.

Criticism of conference proceedings and the type of meetings that give rise to these little-loved tomes is not a new phenomenom. But denigrate them as we will, the medico-scientific jumbo conferences still have their following - attracting many who have a remote interest in the subject but a great interest in the selected venue, which they visit thoroughly - and the sessions sporadically, if at all. There are smaller versions of the jumbo, where the participants are expected to play some role, so their attitude is more serious and their attendance at sessions more faithful.

Fortunately for the rest of us the round table by invitation has increased in popularity during the last 10 years. The small number of participants at the round table, hand picked by the organisers for their expertise and willingness to communicate, does tend to produce a meeting that interests and stimulates the other invitees, and may even achieve some goals as a result of time spent together.

Such a round table meeting was that on which this book is based. The imprint of its convener and organiser, Olga Genbačev, was clear on every aspect, and whatever success in its aims was achieved is due to her direction and enthusiasm. Those who attended the meeting tried to put into their contributions some of her enthusiasm in the search for more knowledge and improved use of the knowledge we already have. Her fellow editors have tried to make a reflection of this spirit apparent in this book. Together we chose the topics, the participants, and the format of this publication. And any faults that arise from this freedom are ours alone - for scientists are not without prejudices and irrationality.

Most forewords end with pious hopes, and this one will be no exception. The hopes are simply that the placenta - until now imperfectly understood and too little used - will become the standard model for appropriate studies, and used as a source of the many valuable substances it appears to contain.

Both these hopes can be realised if at least some of the work described in the pages that follow proceeds to its logical conclusion.

Rebecca Beaconsfield
London

ACKNOWLEDGEMENTS

We would like to thank the Director of the Institute of Endocrinology, Immunology and Nutrition (INEP), Dr. M. Movsesijan, for offering us hospitality, and members of the Institute's staff for their willing help and innumerable courtesies which contributed so much to the success and enjoyment of the meeting.

We also wish to record our thanks to Miss Vera Vujadinović for dealing so efficiently and cheerfully with the secretarial work and the technical problems of a meeting planned and taking place entirely in English in a non-English speaking country.

CONTENTS

PLACENTA AS A SOURCE

GENERAL INTRODUCTION

The placenta is a constant source of wonder to those who study it. The profligacy of nature in creating a structure that possesses so many of the functions of a whole organism, but which has a total life span of only nine months seems an amazing extravagance. In addition to being a microcosm, as Peter Beaconsfield aptly described it many years ago, it has its own specific and individual activity, and functions with less instruction than any other organ of the body.

Recent appreciation of the self-regulatory nature of the placenta casts a new light on the integration of body functions. As regards its endocrine role, much of the material in this book supports the growing realisation that the placenta is autonomous, the release of its characteristic hormones such as chorionic gonadotrophin being governed by autocrine signals from within the trophoblast, or at most by paracrine signals from adjacent tissue, such as the endometrium. Maintenance of normal pregnancy is probably owed to such regulation, and extension of this knowledge could throw light on many problems - faulty implantation, with all its consequences, among them.

It is in the study of this early stage, when clinical malformations begin, that gaps exist in our knowledge and our experimental possibilities. Choriovillous sampling may provide for this need in the future. In the meantime, we can gain insight into disorders of placental function using existing *in vitro* models. An essential prerequisite is to explore the mechanics of their operation and even more importantly to define their limitations.

There is no universal model; all have their limitations. It would be unfortunate if the placenta were to share the fate of many excellent models now discarded because they failed to give results when used in studies for which they were unsuitable.

Tissue culture, cell culture, and whole and part organ perfusion can be carried out on the placenta, and the results of these different studies compared - for the same organ. No other human tissue lends itself to this kind of parallel investigation.

What can the individual expertise of people working on the placenta and on aspects of local regulation contribute to building up a composite picture for each other, the clinician, and the patient?

This question provided the motive for holding a meeting - the meeting on which this book is based. The participants were invited to contribute on the basis of what they thought their work might add to present knowledge as well as to try to clarify some well recognised problems.

How satisfactorily these aims were achieved, and whether they are well presented in this slightly unusual format, is for the reader to judge. We have eschewed making a book that is the proceedings of a meeting, because we feel it is high time the mould of "proceedings" books was broken. Such books decorate the shelves of those who attend the meeting but rarely do they, or anyone else, refer to them.

The usual device of faithfully recording, in dialogue format, the exchange of often banal comments after the presentation of each paper - euphemistically referred to as "Discussion" - has been scrapped. Instead, the editors have tried to distill the salient points of what was presented - inevitably overlaid by our own prejudices - in a form that we hope will be acceptable and informative to any reader. This has taken the form of a post hoc editorial comment in the first section, intended to give our view of the discussion, which ranged well beyond question and answer, and editorial introductions to the second and third sections sketching in some relevant background. We hope to interest our readers and encourage them to speculate on the meaning of the findings. Experience has shown that merely to pile up data in the Micawberish hope that "something will turn up" is a futile exercise.

It is our belief that people from a variety of scientific disciplines will find material of interest in this book, whether or not their major interest is the placenta. Ideas presented here may provoke further work, or complement what is already in progress. If we simply make the reader think, it will fulfil a part of what scientific get-togethers are supposed to be all about.

As scientists we cannot adopt the bureaucrat's panacea for all administrative ills - ignore them, in the hope that they may go away. On the contrary, we know that every new piece of knowledge brings in its train a new group of problems. The use of the placenta in an ever-widening variety of experimental exercises seems to offer tremendous scope of a novel kind in tackling some of these.

PERFUSION OF THE PLACENTA

PROTEIN RELEASE BY THE *IN VITRO* HUMAN PLACENTAL LOBULE WHEN DUALLY PERFUSED

BY DIFFERENT PROTOCOLS

K.R. Page, D.R. Abramovich, C.G. Dacke, K. Henderson and A. Klopper

University of Aberdeen, Marischal College, Aberdeen

Alone of the *in vitro* methods of studying placental function, the dually-perfused placenta preserves the integrity of the fetal and maternal circulations so allowing studies of the "sidedness" of the organ, a point of particular relevance to feto-maternal endocrine physiology. Difficulties in studying the whole human placenta arise from the problems of obtaining a complete, uninjured specimen, and in maintaining adequate perfusion of the entire intervillous space. These difficulties may be minimised by perfusing a limited region of the placenta only, typically a lobule of 25 g wet weight.[1] Lobules selected for this purpose are each supplied by a single fetal artery and vein which may be cannulated from the fetal surface. The maternal aspect is perfused by glass cannulae inserted into the lobular intervillous space, the outflow being collected by drainage from the maternal plate. The perfusate is a physiologically balanced solution such as Earle's culture medium, Medium 199, or Krebs Ringer containing either albumin or Dextran. Perfusions can be maintained for three to 12 hours.

Using this technique it has been shown[2] that over an 80-minute period progesterone is released from both sides of the lobule while human chorionic gonadotrophin (hCG) and human placental lactogen (hPL) are released into the maternal perfusate only. Perfusate was passed once only through the lobule (open circuit) and a marked fall in protein release occurred during the first 20 minutes. The initial release was attributed to secretion of previously synthesised protein. Changes in protein content between perfused and unperfused tissues added to the accumulated protein content of the perfusates led the authors to conclude that net protein synthesis had occurred. This result has been supported by others subsequently.[3,4] Closed circuit methods were employed,[4] and perfusate in both circulations was continuously recycled between tissue and reservoirs (120 ml total volume in each circuit). Evidence for net protein synthesis of hCG, hPL, Schwangerschaftsprotein 1 (SP1) and pregnancy associated plasma protein A (PAPP-A) was obtained over perfusion periods of four hours using Earle's solution gassed with 95% O_2 and 5% CO_2. Tissue levels of all four pregnancy-associated proteins remained remarkably constant throughout perfusion whereas tissue contents of the non-placental proteins haemoglobin (Hb), prolactin, and pregnancy-associated α_2 glycoprotein (α_2-PEG) all showed significant falls. Likewise tissue levels of all four placental proteins fell when the perfusate contained the protein synthesis inhibitors cycloheximide or puromycin, or the metabolic inhibitors iodoacetic acid or 2,4-dinitrophenol. However, corresponding changes in protein release into perfusate were less well defined in these experiments.

15

Release of newly synthesised protein into maternal plasma is affected by a number of factors. Apart from membrane events at the microvillous border, diffusion across the unstirred layer of solution immediately adjacent to the trophoblast may be of importance. The proteins will have low free solution diffusion coefficients and in consequence this unstirred layer might become rate controlling. The effect will be compounded by inadequacies of the *in vitro* method of perfusion. In life the placental intervillous space develops in association with the maternal spiral arteries. However careful the cannulation it is highly unlikely *in vitro* perfusion can mimic exactly the flow pattern produced by these spiral arteries.

Inadequacies in lobule perfusion may also arise from a variety of other causes. It is impossible to restrict maternal perfusate to the region receiving fetal perfusion.[5] Maternal perfusate will thus come into contact with a greater volume of tissue than the dually perfused lobule. Tissue not receiving fetal perfusate will be in poorer condition, and consequently cell death may be higher in extralobular regions with consequent effects on the solute levels in the maternal outflow. Even within regions of dual perfusion pockets of unperfused tissue can persist. As much as a third of both fetal vascular space and maternal intervillous space may remain unperfused.[6] We have observed surges of protein release during perfusion, and believe these may come from unperfused regions of the lobule opening up after the start of perfusion.[7]

This paper will therefore attempt to evaluate how far protein release into maternal perfusate accurately reflects protein synthesis in placental trophoblast. Results to be discussed were all obtained using the methods described by Abramovich and colleagues.[5] The placenta was mounted with the maternal surface dependent and standard flow rates of 6 ml/min fetal and 20 ml/min mataral side were used. All solutions were gassed with 95% O_2 and 5% CO_2 and in closed circuit perfusate volumes of 140 ml were employed. All placentae were obtained from normal term deliveries (vaginal or elective Caesarean section) and fully perfused within 15 to 30 minutes of delivery.

PROTEIN RELEASE UNDER CONTINUOUS OPEN CIRCUIT (Protocol A)

In order to establish the time course of protein release into maternal perfusate, placentae were perfused under open circuit conditions for periods of 220 minutes. Krebs-Ringer containing 3% Dextran (60 KD) was used. Outflows were collected at 10-minute periods from both circuits, the volume recorded and 5 ml retained for protein analysis. Experiments were conducted on six placentae. Release of SP_1, hCG, PAPP-A, and hPL occurred on the maternal side of the lobule only. To obtain a relation between the disparate units used in measuring proteins the protein content in each maternal sample was expressed as a percentage of the total protein released in 220 minutes. Results for SP_1, hCG, PAPP-A and hPL (Fig. 1) indicated all four proteins followed a similar time course with a substantial decline in the rate of protein release over the first 100 minutes of perfusion.

PROTEIN RELEASE UNDER ALTERNATE PERIODS OF OPEN AND CLOSED CIRCUIT (Protocols B1, B2 and C)

In these experiments the role of diffusion on protein release rates was examined by perfusing the lobule with Krebs Ringer (protocols B1, B2) or Medium 199 (protocol C), under a repeating cycle of open and closed circuits. Perfusates contained 3% Dextran. In all protocols the lobule was initially perfused under open circuit for 15 minutes and then closed for three consecutive periods of 45 minutes, each period being separated from the other by a 15-minute period of open circuit. Fresh 140 ml volumes of perfusate were used on each closed circuit, perfusates being recovered at the end of each period of open or closed circuit. After measurement of the

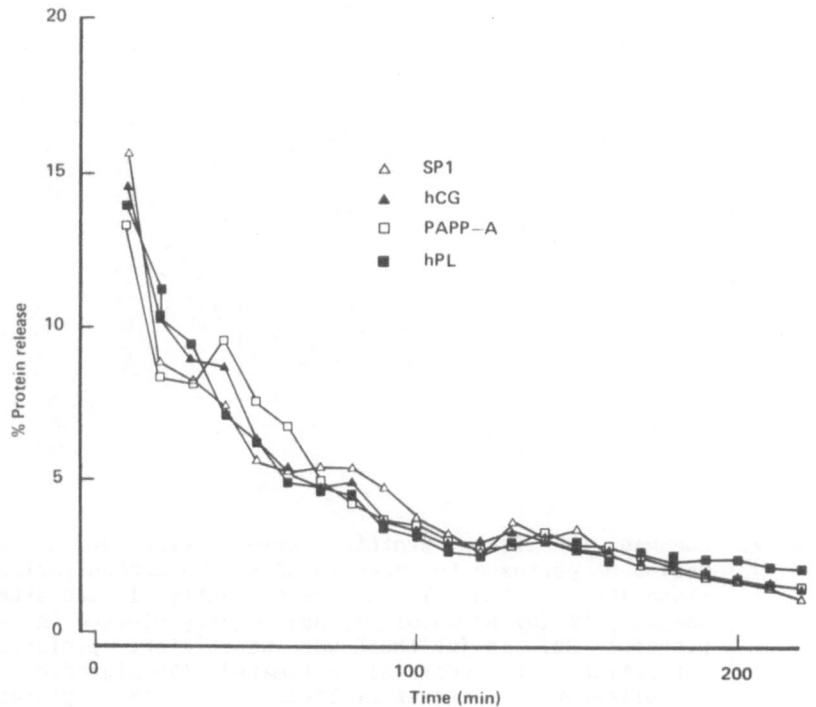

Figure 1.   Points represent protein release over 10 min expres-
             sed as a percentage of the total released in 220 min.
             Each point is the mean from six placentae.

total sample volume 5 ml of each sample was retained for protein and
steroid analysis. Three samples each of perfused and unperfused tissue were
taken from the placenta at the end of the experiment. Each piece of tissue
was blotted between two sheets of thick absorbent paper, using light
pressure in protocols B1 and C, and heavy pressure (in order to remove as
much intervillous fluid as possible) in protocol B2, and then weighed. Both
tissue and perfusate samples were frozen directly and stored at -20° C
until assay. Placental tissue (1 to 2 g) was homogenised with volumes of
ice cold Tris-Cl, centrifuged, and the clear supernatant taken for assay.

Analysis of the tissue samples confirmed previous reports[3,4] in that
levels of pregnancy-associated proteins remained relatively constant with
perfusion, whereas non-trophoblastic proteins showed significant falls
(Figs. 2a,b and 4a). The ratios of perfused to unperfused tissue protein
content of SP_1, hCG, and PAPP-A was significantly higher than that for
prolactin in protocol B1. In protocol B2 prolactin levels in both perfused
and unperfused tissues were too low to provide accurate ratios. In this
protocol, however, the albumin ratio was significantly smaller than those
of the four pregnancy proteins. With respect to the steroids the progesterone ratio was significantly greater than 1 while that of oestradiol (E_2)
was the same as albumin.

While albumin, progesterone, and E_2 were released on both sides of the
placenta SP_1, hCG, PAPP-A, and hPL were released from the maternal side of
the lobule only. Protein release rates were found to be higher under open
circuit conditions than when circuits were closed (Figs. 3, 4b). The level
of protein per g of unperfused tissue was compared to the amount of protein
released to perfusate/gramme of perfused tissue. Tissue to perfusate

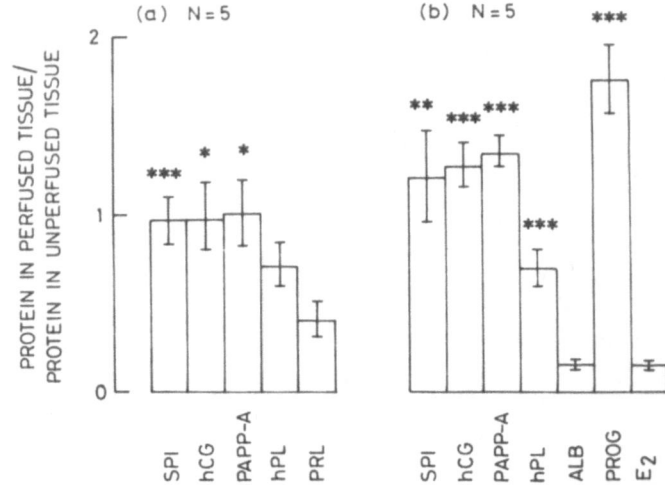

Figure 2. Changes in tissue protein content with perfusion.
Ratios of perfused to unperfused tissue concentrations
shown (Means ± SEM). Tissues were lightly blotted after
sampling in (a) protocol B1, and heavily blotted in (b)
protocol B2. In (b) there was insufficient prolactin
for ratios to be accurately estimated. The significance
of differences between prolactin and other protein
ratios (a) and albumin and other protein ratios (b) is
indicated * P < 0.05 ** P < 0.02 *** P < 0.01 (2 sample
t test).

composition was in the order hPL > hCG > SP_1 > PAPP-A (Tables I and II),
and hPL, hCG, and SP_1 tissue levels correlated significantly with perfusate
composition. No major difference in protein release was observed between
protocols B1 and C.

Table I. Total protein release compared to protein content in
unperfused tissue - protocol B2

Protein	*Tissue content as % of protein release	Correlation coefficient	▪Significance
SP_1	21.3	0.90	*
hCG	26.3	0.96	**
PAPP-A	6.1	-0.23	NS
hPL	106.9	0.93	*

* Tissue content and protein release compared per g wet weight of
unperfused and perfused tissue respectively
▪ ** P < 0.01 * P < 0.05

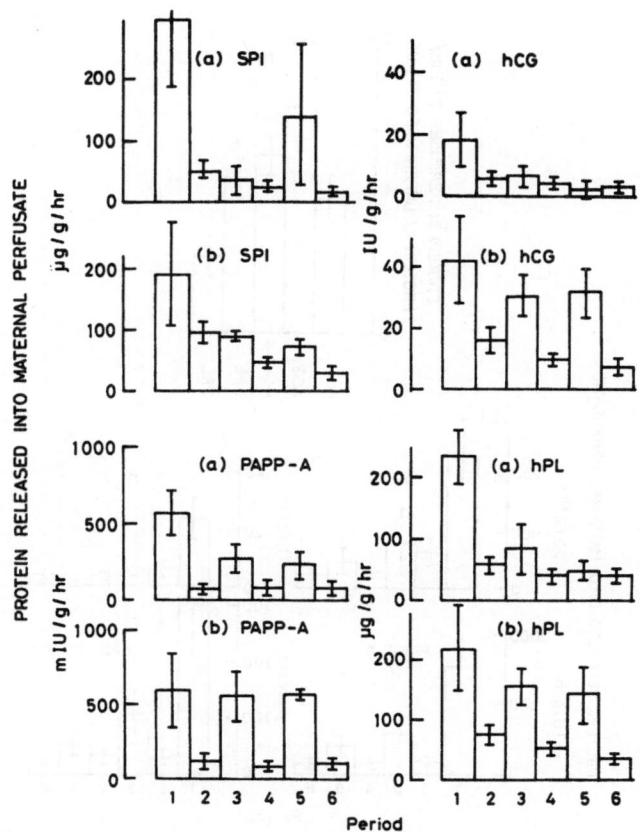

Figure 3. Protein released into maternal perfusate (Krebs Ringer). Means ± SEM shown. (a) and (b) as in Fig. 1. Periods 1 to 6 indicate three successive cycles of open circuit (15 min) followed by closed circuit (45 min).

Table II. Net protein production in 3 hr : data from protocols B1 and C

Protein	Protocol	Perfusate release	Tissue content		Net protein production
			Perfused	Unperfused	
SP$_1$	B1	177.8 ± 60.6	28.7 ± 10.4	28.2 ± 8.6	178.2 ± 58.8
µg/g	C	147.9 ± 68.1	21.3 ± 9.0	20.8 ± 8.1	148.4 ± 68.6
hCG	B1	14480 ± 6470	4116 ± 1553	3808 ± 1432	15790 ± 7060
mIU/g	C	14460 ± 5250	2503 ± 990	1807 ± 878	15160 ± 5210
PAPP-A	B1	419.6 ± 111.6	38.6 ± 12.1	35.1 ± 6.1	423.2 ± 1145
IU/g	C	553.0 ± 162	53.8 ± 9.7	38.5 ± 7.7	568.4 ± 161.4
hPL	B1	187.4 ± 42.7	34.3 ± 19.0	80.1 ± 51.3	141.4 ± 58.4
µg/g	C	233.0 ± 57.3	31.9 ± 27.7	28.1 ± 24.0	236.8 ± 59.6

Means ± SEM shown. Protocol B1 n = 5, Protocol C n = 4.

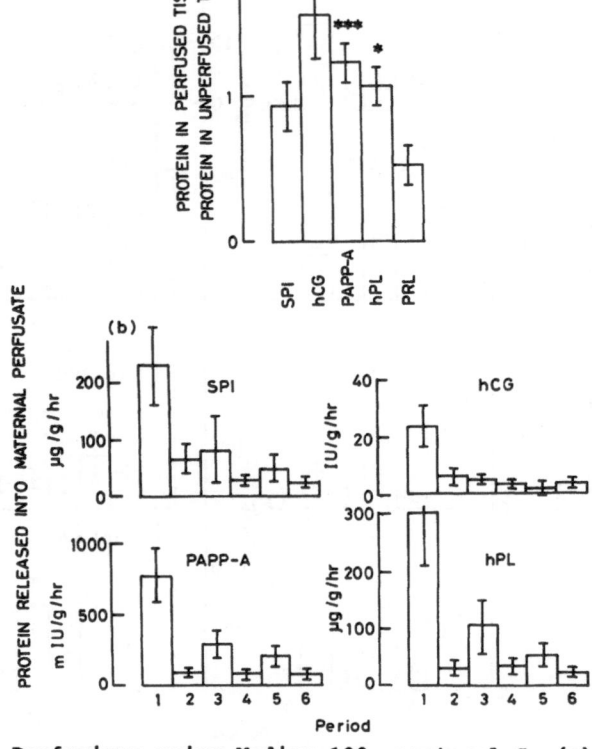

Figure 4.   Perfusions using Medium 199, protocol C. (a) Changes in
tissue protein content. Ratios of perfused to unperfused tissue concentrations shown (Means ± SEM)
and differences relative to prolactin (2 sample t test)
* P < 0.05, *** P < 0.01.

CONCLUSIONS

The presence of albumin, progesterone, and E_2 in perfusate outflows on
both sides of the placenta and the restriction of SP_1, hCG, PAPP-A, hPL,
and prolactin to maternal outflow indicated the physiological properties of
the placental barrier were maintained. The absence of any significant
reduction in tissue content of progesterone, SP_1, hCG, PAPP-A and hPL after
three hours of perfusion contrasted with the marked falls in E_2, albumin
and prolactin. Taken with the observations of other workers[4] about the
effects of inhibitors of either protein synthesis or metabolism on tissue
protein content this provides encouraging evidence for the continuing
synthesis of the four pregnancy-associated proteins.

The consistency of SP_1, hCG, PAPP-A, and hPL tissue levels over a
period of three hours indicates there was no substantial release of
proteins by cell death. Release of K^+ from the perfused lobule is known to
be small,[5] again indicating there is little cell death over this time
period.

The absence of any major differences in results obtained using
protocols B1 and C indicated that within the time scale of these

experiments there was no major effect on protein production that could be attributed to the presence of amino acids in the perfusion fluid. The most important finding regarding protein release was the observation that release rates are significantly higher under open circuit than when circuits are closed. The reversibility of this phenomenon plus the fact it was most marked in the case of PAPP-A, the protein of highest molecular weight, indicated that it arose from a process of diffusion. Under closed circuit conditions the accumulation of protein in the perfusion fluid will reduce the concentration differential between tissue and perfusate and hence lower any diffusive flux of protein.

In the absence of cell death proteins will not be able to diffuse across the microvillous membrane of the syncytiotrophoblast. The most obvious explanation for release by diffusion is to postulate the existence of an unstirred volume of perfusate within the intervillous space. Figure 1 indicates there is a rapid decline in the rate of protein release during the first 100 minutes of perfusion. If the rate of protein entry into the unstirred volume declines faster than the exit of protein by diffusion into the well stirred region of the intervillous space then observed protein release into the perfusate will obey diffusion kinetics. In this situation the protein release to the perfusate will only reflect the membrane processes when the system approaches a steady state – that is, when protein entry into the unstirred space matches release into the well stirred perfusate.

If such an unstirred volume exists then it is possible all the protein released into the perfusate is preformed protein trapped in the intervillous space prior to the start of perfusion. There are two lines of reasoning which show that this is not the case. The first examines the mass balance of protein production. This is shown for protocols B1 and C in Table II. In these protocols tissues were only lightly blotted prior to assay and so would retain much of the intervillous fluid. The Table shows perfusate release greatly exceeded changes in tissue composition for all four trophoblastic proteins. The second compares total protein release to the amount of protein contained in the lobular intervillous space when filled with maternal plasma. This last (i.v.s. plasma protein) is estimated as the product of intervillous volume (obtained from lobular wet weight and the weight to volume relationship[8]) and the protein concentrations shown in Table III. Figure 5 shows the ratio of total protein release to i.v.s. plasma protein ranges from 5 for SP_1 to 124 for hPL.

Although the intervillous plasma will have a higher protein concentration than peripheral blood,[9] the difference is not sufficient to explain these ratios, so once again it can be concluded protein release is greatly in excess of material trapped in the intervillous space before perfusion.

The ratios in Figure 5 suggest a protein release rate in the order hPL > PAPP-A > hCG > SP_1. Figure 6 shows both open and closed circuit releases of hPL, PAPP-A, and hCG increase with time in relation to release of SP_1. The low release rate of SP_1 contrasts with its high concentration in maternal plasma compared to hPL. However, it should be noted it has a much longer plasma half life than hPL (Table III).

Although the kinetics of protein release indicate the presence of an unstirred volume its physical nature cannot be determined at present. As outlined earlier there is evidence that the intervillous space is not uniformly perfused.[6,7] Material will also enter the maternal perfusate from regions that receive no fetal perfusion.[5] There will be an "unstirred layer" immediately adjacent to the microvillous border of the trophoblast and this may be accentuated by pockets formed in the plasmalemma by fused exocytotic vesicles. All these phenomena will contribute to an effective unstirred volume.

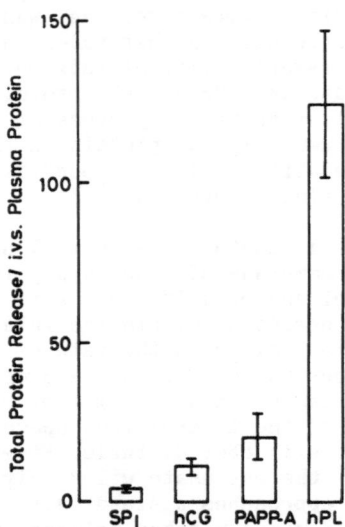

Figure 5.   Total protein release divided by the protein contained
in lobular intervillous space when filled with plasma
of composition shown in Table III.   Means ± SEM. Data
from protocol B2 (n = 5).

Table III. Protein concentrations and plasma half-lifes (data obtained
using protocol B2)

	SP₁ μg/ml	hCG IU/ml	PAPP-A IU/ml	hPL μg/ml
Maternal plasma	150.0	13.0	100.0	6
*Unperfused tissue	45.5	12.2	52.4	264
ˤPerfusate period 1	3.4	0.8	10.3	4
*Perfused tissue	52.8	15.4	59.0	172
ˤPerfusate period 6	2.5	0.7	9.8	3
Maternal plasma half-life (hr)	20-40	–	–	0.25-0.30

* Concentration per g wet weight

ˤ Period 1 is the first 15 min period of open circuit and period 6 is
the last 45 min period of closed circuit.

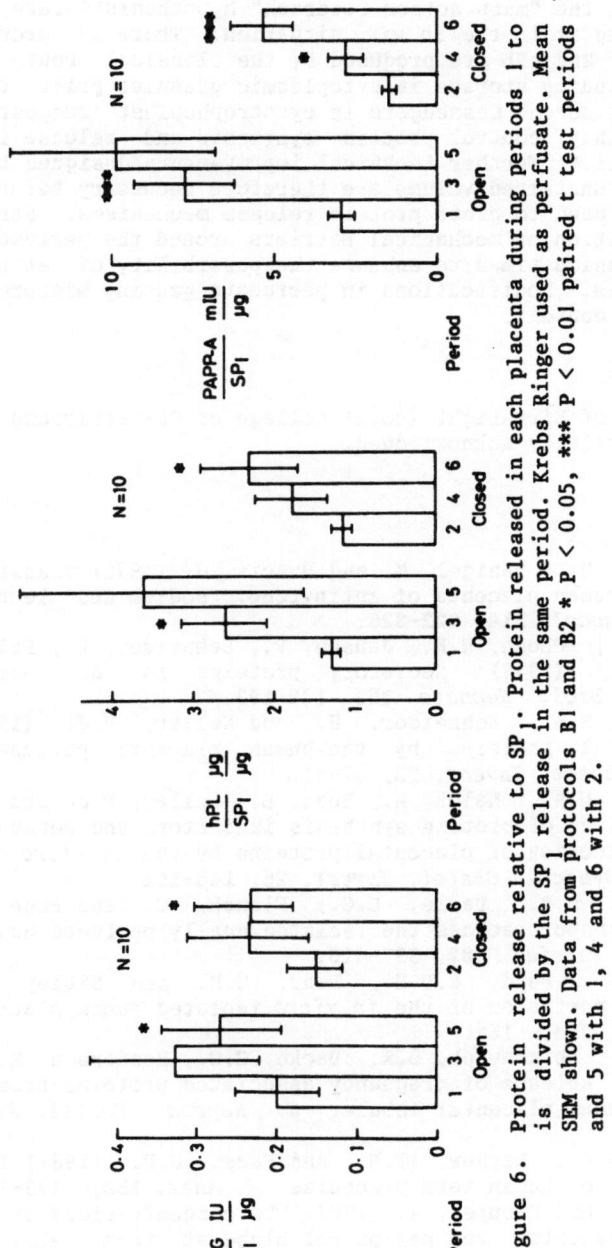

Figure 6. Protein released in each placenta during periods 1 to 6 is divided by the SP_1 release in the same period. Krebs Ringer used as perfusate. Mean $\pm \frac{1}{3}$ SEM shown. Data from protocols B1 and B2 * $P < 0.05$, *** $P < 0.01$ paired t test periods 5 with 1, 4 and 6 with 2.

The dually perfused lobule will therefore exaggerate the role of diffusion in protein release. Not only will perfusion of intervillous space be less efficient than in life, but the concentration gradients will be larger owing to the low protein levels in the perfusate (apart from hPL) compared with *in vivo* plasma levels (Table III). Thus although the present results fit well the "mass action feedback" hypothesis[10] care must be taken in extrapolating it to the *in vivo* situation. There is growing evidence that both hCG and hPL are produced by the classical route for protein synthesis including storage in cytoplasmic granules prior to release.[11] The presence of second messengers in cytotrophoblast suggests mechanisms may be present that control protein synthesis and release in response to external stimuli.[12] Further technical improvements designed to reduce the effects of the unstirred volume are therefore necessary before the model can reliably be used to probe protein release mechanisms. Strategies could include the addition of mechanical barriers around the perfused lobule and extending perfusion times to enhance the possibility of attaining steady state conditions. Modifications in perfusate gassing mixtures[13] could be helpful in this context.

Acknowledgements

The support of Birthright (Royal College of Obstetricians and Gynaecologists) is gratefully acknowledged.

REFERENCES

1. Schneider, H., Panigel, M. and Dancis, J. (1972) Transfer across the perfused human placenta of antipyrene, sodium and leucine. *Am. J. Obstet. Gynecol.* **114**, 822–828.
2. Dancis, J., Ghosh, N.K., Jansen, V., Schneider, H., Fallon, R.J. and Cox, R.P. (1979) Secretory proteins in the perfused human placenta. *Biol. Neonate* **35**, 188–193.
3. Bersinger, N.A., Schneider, H. and Keller, P.J. (1986) Synthesis of placental proteins by the human placenta perfused *in vitro*. *Gynecol. Obstet. Invest.* **22**, 47–51.
4. Bersinger, N.A., Malek, A., Benz, B., Keller, P.J. and Schneider, H. (1988) Effect of protein synthesis inhibitors and metabolic blockers on the production of placental proteins by the *in vitro* perfused human placenta. *Gynecol. Obstet. Invest.* **25**, 145–151.
5. Abramovich, D.R., Dacke, C.G., Elcock, C. and Page, K.R. (1987) Calcium transport across the isolated dually perfused human placental lobule. *J. Physiol.* **382**, 397–410.
6. Barker, G., Boyd, R.D.H., Lear, G.H. and Sibley, C.P. (1987) Incomplete perfusion of the *in vitro* isolated human placental lobule. *J. Physiol.* **394**, 168.
7. Page, K.R., Abramovich, D.R., Dacke, C.G., Henderson, K. and Klopper, A. (1988) Release of pregnancy-associated proteins from the dually perfused human placental lobule. *J. Reprod. Fertil. Suppl.* **36**, 184–185.
8. Jackson, M.R., Mayhew, T.M. and Haas, J.D. (1987) The volumetric composition of human term placentae. *J. Anat.* **152**, 173–187.
9. Ahmed, A.G. and Klopper, A. (1983) The concentrations of SP$_1\beta$ and SP$_1\alpha$ in retroplacental and peripheral blood at term. *Eurp. J. Obstet. Gynecol. Reprod. Biol.* **16**, 77–81.
10. Chard T. (1986) Placental syntheses. *Clin. Obstet. Gynecol.* **13**, 447–467.
11. Johnson, S.A. and Wooding, F.B.P. (1988) Synthesis and storage of chorionic gonadotrophin and placental lactogen in human syncytiotrophoblast. *J. Physiol. Soc.* **44**, 50.
12. Feinman, M.A., Kliman, H.J., Caltabiano, S.E. and Strauss, J.F. (1986) 8-Bromo-3',5'-Adenosine monophosphate stimulates the endocrine

activity of human cytotrophoblasts in culture. *J. Clin. Endocrinol. Metab.* **63**, 1211-1217.

13. Miller, R.K., Weir, P.J., Maulik, D. and di Sant'Agnese P.A. (1985) Human placenta *in vitro* : characterisation during 12 hr of dual perfusion. *Contrib. Gynecol. Obstet.* **13**, 77-84.

CRITERIA FOR *IN VITRO* DUAL PERFUSIONS IN THE HUMAN PLACENTAL LOBULE: PERFUSIONS IN EXCESS OF 12 HOURS

Richard K. Miller,[1] Patrick J. Wier,[2] Yogesh Shah,[1] P.A. di Sant'Agnese[1] and Rogelio Perez D'Gregorio[3]

Rochester, NY,[1] King of Prussia, PA,[2] USA; Caracas,[3] Venezuela

To study the normal functions of the human chorioallantoic placenta as well as the influence of xenobiotics, one *in vitro* technique alone allows the investigator to examine haemodynamics, transplacental transport, cellular uptake, endocrine function, and metabolism – dual perfusion of the isolated human placenta. This chapter will concentrate on the use of the *in vitro* dual perfusion of the human placenta for periods beyond the four hours used by the majority of investigators.

Perfusion of the human placenta has been carried out under different conditions: maternal only,[1] fetal only,[2] and dual. Since the early work on dual perfusion of the entire human placenta *in vitro* [3,4] numerous investigators have worked to improve conditions for *in vitro* perfusion of the whole placenta.[5-11] While dual perfusion of the whole placenta may best represent the situation in utero, the technique is limited by the need for a placenta which is intact. It has been estimated that only 10% of placentas delivered can be used for whole organ perfusion. For this reason, investigators have been most successful with perfusion of a portion of the human placenta corresponding to a cotyledon or lobule.[12,13] Currently, human placental perfusions are limited to third trimester tissue because of the damage to villi during delivery of earlier organs.

Figure 1 is a diagram of a typical circuit. The fetal circulation is established by cannulation of a single chorionic artery and its companion vein supplying a placental lobule, which is usually peripheral, though central lobules can also be used. The overlapping intervillous space is perfused by at least two cannulae piercing the decidual surface. The venous outflow of the intervillous space is through openings in the decidual plate. The perfused lobule (approximately 25 g) is isolated from the remainder of the placenta by clamping the surrounding tissue between a plastic gasket and supporting base. There have been a number of adaptations of the perfusion model from having the maternal/decidual surface position superior – the most usual – to having the decidual surface directed downward so that the maternal perfusate drips from the placental surface and is collected in a funnel.[14-16] Depending on the requirements of the study, the maternal and fetal circuits may be "open" (no recirculation of perfusate) or "closed" (with recirculation of perfusate). An open system may be preferable when examining the transfer of compounds using clearance ratios, since it is important to have no compound in the fetal arterial circulation; however, to determine accurately changes in fetal volume, the

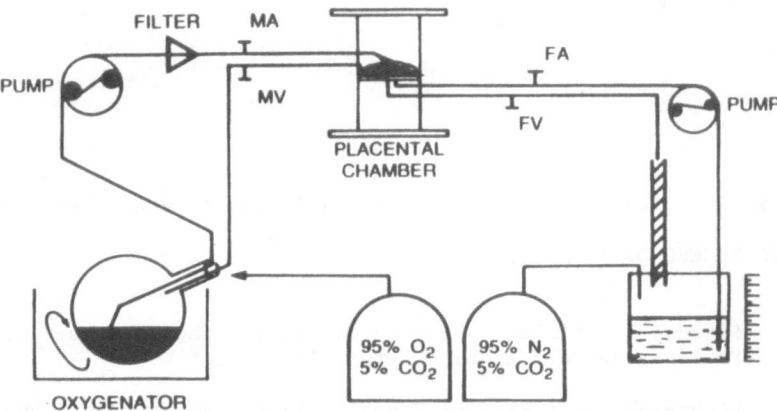

Figure 1.   Schematic diagram of the perfusion apparatus for iso-
             lated dual perfusion of the human placental lobule. MA
             = Maternal artery; MV = Maternal vein; FA = Fetal
             artery; FV = Fetal vein. Not shown are the water baths
             used to maintain both reservoirs and the placental
             chamber at 37° C. Also not shown are the two humidi-
             fiers for the gas mixture.

production of small quantities of placental constituents – for example,
placental proteins – or for prolonged perfusions (> 2 hrs) a closed or
recirculating system for both maternal and fetal perfusates is preferable.
There is considerable flexibility in the way the perfusion system can be
used, and therefore during the course of an experiment both open and closed
systems may be used.

Fluids which have been used for human placental perfusion include
balanced salt solutions (Earle's, Ringer's, or Krebs-Ringer-phosphate
bicarbonate) containing glucose (1.0–1.5 mg/ml) and low molecular weight
Dextran (20–40 mg/ml), or serum albumin (1–20 mg/ml) with additions of
essential amino-acids.[15,17-19] Even whole human blood or red blood cells
in various proportions have been added to the balanced salt solutions in
hopes of producing better survival.[20-25]

Investigators have now turned to developing a perfusion model which
will provide normal data for extended periods of time. For success in
perfusing a human placental lobule it is essential to allow the tissue to
recover from the trauma of delivery and ischaemia, which usually takes
about an hour; to establish adequate base line data and be sure the
preparation is functioning properly (usually one hour); and only then
conduct the experimental protocol under study.

If these requirements are to be met then prolonged perfusion (> 2
hours) of the placenta is needed to study the placental transfer of
molecules which pass slowly through the placenta, as well as hormone
synthesis and toxic interactions.

LONG-TERM PERFUSION

To meet the needs of extended *in vitro* perfusion, a synthetic tissue
culture medium (M199) providing essential amino acids, vitamins, co-
factors, nucleosides, and intermediary metabolites is necessary.[26] Further

to improve perfusion and to supply sufficient oxygen, maternal perfusates have been equilibrated with 95% oxygen and 5% carbon dioxide, and fetal perfusates equilibrated with 95% nitrogen and 5% carbon dioxide. This achieves a more physiological oxygen tension in the fetal vessels.[27-29] Recent studies have shown that high oxygen tensions supplied to the fetal circuit produce alterations in placental morphology within two hours.[30]

During long-term perfusions both maternal and fetal perfusates are recirculated in order to conserve perfusates. As a consequence of recirculation nutrients are depleted, and metabolic wastes begin to accumulate after about three hours. It is therefore essential to provide both maternal and fetal circulations with fresh perfusates at least every four hours during these prolonged perfusions.[31]

To establish the viability of the preparation measurements must be taken both during the perfusion and after completion of the study (Table I). Among the initial criteria for assessing integrity and function of the perfused preparation are measurements of net transfer of oxygen (maternal to fetal).[27] This measurement confirms the efficiency and overlap of intervillous space and fetal vessel circulations, adequate overlap being a prerequisite for measuring placental transfer *in vitro*. By measuring the oxygen content in all four sampling ports (fetal vein and artery; maternal vein and artery), one can establish quantitatively the degree of perfusion/perfusion overlap achieved. A minimal venous to arterial difference on the fetal side of 60 mm Hg for the pO_2 is essential. This difference in fetal venous-arterial pO_2 is dependent upon a fetal arterial pO_2 of less than 70 mm Hg. If the oxygen values are too low in the fetal vein then repositioning of the maternal catheters can be achieved quickly.

In fact, if the maternal catheters are not in the fetally perfused lobule then the fetal venous pO_2 can be lower than the fetal arterial pO_2.

Among the principal determinants of overall function of the placenta are haemodynamics, metabolism, and morphology. Measurements of fetal capillary resistance (fetal perfusion pressure (> 70 mm Hg)) and permeability (volume maintenance in the fetal circuit (> 2 ml/hr)) are critical for demonstrating the integrity of the fetal vasculature. Equally important

Table I.   Criteria for dual perfusion of the human placenta

During Perfusion:

Perfusion Pressure (fetal vein and artery)
Flow Rate
Fetal Volume Loss (< 2 ml/hr)
pH, pCO_2, pO_2, [HCO_3]
  (Maternal and Fetal)
Oxygen consumption
Net Fetal Oxygen Transfer
Energy Charge

Post Perfusion:

Glucose Utilisation
Lactate Production
Protein Synthesis
Hormone Production/Directional Release
Tissue Content
Tissue Slice Incubation (AIB)
Enzyme Release (LDH)
Morphology - Ultrastructure

29

though is the fetal venous pressure; fetal venous pressures in excess of 20 cm of water have been reported to increase fetal volume loss.[32] In combination with net fetal oxygen transfer, fetal volume loss and fetal pressure/flow rate represent the principal four points of evaluation to establish whether a perfusion can be extended.

In addition to oxygen content measurements, other "marker" substrates - such as tritiated water and antipyrine - can be used to assess the efficiency of intervillous space and fetal capillary perfusion as well as the degree of maternal-fetal perfusion overlap.[32] We have found that these markers are not useful indicators of perfusion/perfusion overlap when compared with net oxygen transfer.[27,28] Since oxygen is consumed by the placenta, its diffusion distance is small; however, for the above molecules they will reach the fetally perfused region eventually and then equilibrate with the fetal circuit, but the time involved may limit the viability of the preparation, not to mention the kinetic analysis involved. By limiting the kinetic analysis, one assumes that the particular molecule under study has the same characteristics as antipyrine or water. However, if the substance is highly lipid soluble - for example, phenytoin and dioxin - the comparison may not be appropriate.[28,33] If the perfusion/perfusion overlap is not close the maternally perfused tissue may concentrate the lipid soluble substance while allowing the antipyrine or water to equilibrate eventually. Therefore, a much larger percentage of the administered test substance may be held in a non-fetally perfused compartment. Similar problems may arise for highly protein bound molecules - for example, dioxin and manganese.[29] With long-term perfusions, there is a fourth compartment - the non-perfused tissue within the chamber. This fourth compartment is filled as fluid diffuses out from the perfusion/perfusion overlap area. Molecules may be preferentially retained in this compartment based upon their interactions with cellular components. Thus, all regions of placental tissue within the perfusion chamber must be monitored.

The most commonly employed indicators of metabolic integrity of perfused placenta are oxygen consumption and glucose consumption/lactate production.[34] For extended perfusions up to 24 hours these values have been among the most stable.

Additional measures of energy charge can now be monitored on a continual basis during a perfusion. Thus, beta-ATP, inorganic phosphorus, and tissue pH can be assessed by undertaking magnetic resonance imaging (MRI) spectra every 20 minutes or less.[35] Until recently, all measurements of ATP and creatine phosphate have required the termination of the experiment to assess tissue content; however, use of magnetic resonance imaging spectroscopy for phosphorus now provides for a continual monitoring of placental energy charge throughout the course of an experiment. Metabolism markers more specific to the placenta are measures of protein hormone (hCG, hPL) synthesis and release (Table II; Fig. 2).[31]

Except for use of MRI spectroscopy to monitor tissue pH and phosphorus content continuously, other methods to assess placental function are restricted to evaluations of perfusate and tissue samples obtained before the start of perfusion or after perfusion. Unfortunately, biopsy sampling of the perfused tissue during the study leads to a dramatic alteration in tissue viability criteria - fetal volume loss, for example.

Equally important monitors of integrity and function are morphological assessments including ultrastructural examination. Unsatisfactory perfusion results initially in syncytiotrophoblast changes such as dilatation of endoplasmic reticulum, loss of microvilli, and appearance of lysosome-like bodies. Later it leads to distortion of mitochondria with pyknosis of syncytial nuclei.[23,36,37] Even when there is excellent overall pre-servation of placental cells villous stromal oedema and slight

Table II.   Rate of placental lactogen (hPL) and chorionic gonadotrophin (hCG) release into the maternal circulation in the dually perfused human placenta following 12 hours of perfusion

Hormone	N[1]	Release Rate	Percent of Control[2]		
		(1-2 hrs)	(2-6 hrs)	(6-10 hrs)	(10-12 hrs)
		ug/min Kg			
hPL	9	555 ± 225	112 ± 31	93 ± 36	87 ± 22
		IU/min Kg			
hCG	9	127 ± 62	104 ± 36	88 ± 20	83 ± 26

[1]   Number of perfusions
[2]   Percent of control, where control is the 1-2 hr value, is calculated as the individual values from each experiment and then averaged

syncytiotrophoblast vesiculation are common artifacts.[38-40] Recent developments in preparation of specimens for both light and ultrastructural examination allows specific areas of the placental tissue to be seen under light microscopy and that specific region "popped off" for ultrastructural viewing.[41, 42] Good preservation of structure can be seen even after 12-18 hours of perfusion. High resolution plastic sections of perfused placentae can give substantial detail (Fig. 3). Stromal oedema and subsyncytiotrophoblastic vesiculations are observed in some instances. However, their severity is distinctly correlated to the amount of fetal volume loss. Oedema may be also related to pre-existing pathology since oedema may also be seen in preperfusion specimens. Electron micrographs of perfused placentae which are "popped off" the plastic sections demonstrate apparently normal structure with excellent preservation of cells (Fig. 4).

Sustained perfusion of the human placental lobule provides many opportunities for investigating the interactions of therapeutic and environmental agents as well as the normal function of the trophoblast. In all these studies, it is clear that perturbing the system is essential to understanding its operation, and having control values for the parameters under study is critical. However, it is equally important to have base line values for other biochemical, physiological, and morphological functions to be sure that the system is operating properly (Table I). As the perfusion model is further developed, better refined and defined evaluations of function will be possible. However, without the types of functions listed in Table I as base line parameters there can be doubts about whether and how well the placenta is functioning.

With such parameters taken as a base line, in depth studies of transport, metabolism and toxic interaction can be carried out. Nutrient transfer by the placenta has been extensively investigated with *in vitro* perfusion, but few studies have examined the transport of substances for more than two hours. For some nutrients, such as vitamin B_{12}, little

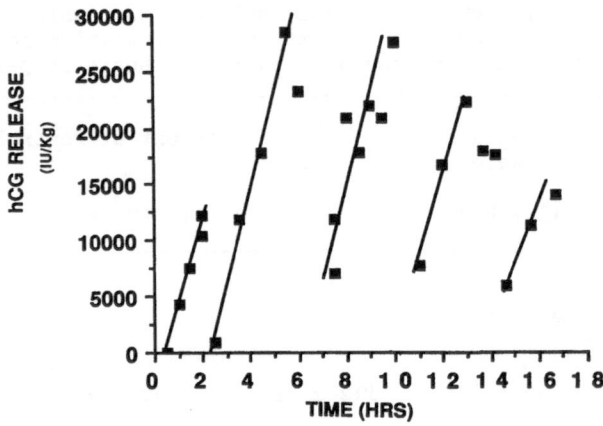

Figure 2.   Release of human chorionic gonadotrophin (hCG) into the
maternal circuit during 18 hrs of dual perfusion.

Transfusions of maternal and fetal perfusates occurred
at 2 hrs and then at 4 hr-intervals; thereafter. In
this experiment the initial rates of hCG release did
not differ significantly during the perfusion. A similar pattern was noted for human placental lactogen
release. However, in other experiments, when a reduction in the release of one hormone appeared, there was
a similar reduction in the release of the other. These
changes all occurred with a maintenance of oxygen
consumption and glucose utilisation. In nearly, but not
all, instances there was also an increase in fetal
volume loss (> 4 ml/hr). Also noted in this figure is a
commonly found decrease in the amount of protein
hormone actually circulating in the maternal perfusate
after multiple hours of perfusion. Such a decrease is
not due to increased net transfer to the fetal circuit,
nor simply a decrease in release. Rather this decrease
in circulating hormone (hCG or hPL) is most likely
associated with catabolism or accumulation by the
placenta itself. The feedback of hCG on protein synthesis by the perfused placenta has not been investigated
to date. Thus, this curiosity of decreasing levels of
placentally produced protein hormones is reproducible,
but unexplained. When the placental tissues are analysed at the termination of the experiment, the levels of
hCG and hPL are comparable.

vitamin is actually transferred from mother to conceptus within two to
three hours. Measurable quantities of the vitamin cross after four
hours.[43,44]

    Movement of viruses across the placenta can be tracked during extended
perfusions. In one study substantial amounts of echo 11 and coxsackie B
viruses were recovered from the placental lobule, but none from fetal
circuit even after 15 hours.[45]

Table III.   Effects of cycloheximide on the release of human chorionic gonadotrophin into the maternal circulation and tissue content of the dually perfused human placenta

hCG Release

Xenobiotic	N^1	Percent of Control[2] at 5 - 8 hours
Cycloheximide[3,4] $(10^{-4}$ M)	3	15 ± 6

Tissue Content of hCG

Xenobiotic	N^1	Fresh IU/Gm	Percent Perfused/Fresh[5]
Control	9	24 ± 5	96 ± 5
Cycloheximide[3,4] $(10^{-4}$ M)	3	22 ± 6	$18 \pm 2*$

[1]   Number of placental perfusions
[2]   Percent of control, where control is the initial time period before addition of xenobiotic, is calculated as the individual values from each experiment and then averaged
[3]   The concentrations of xenobiotic represent initial concentrations of xenobiotic. No additional xenobiotic was added at subsequent transfusions
[4]   Experiments terminated at < 8 hrs following addition of xenobiotic due to fetal volume loss > 5 ml/hr
[5]   Percent perfused/fresh is calculated as the individual values in each experiment and then averaged
* $p < 0.05$. Mean $\pm$ SD

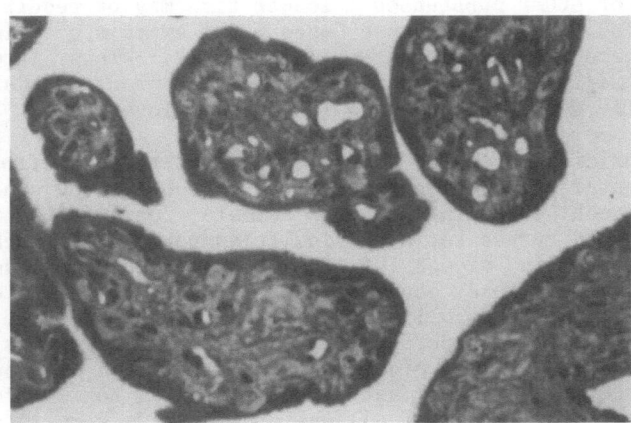

Figure 3.   Twelve-hour perfused placental lobule with no significant morphological alterations except for relatively increased number of cytotrophoblast cells. Note absence of red blood cells (Spurr plastic, basic fuchsin-methylene blue x 300).[40]

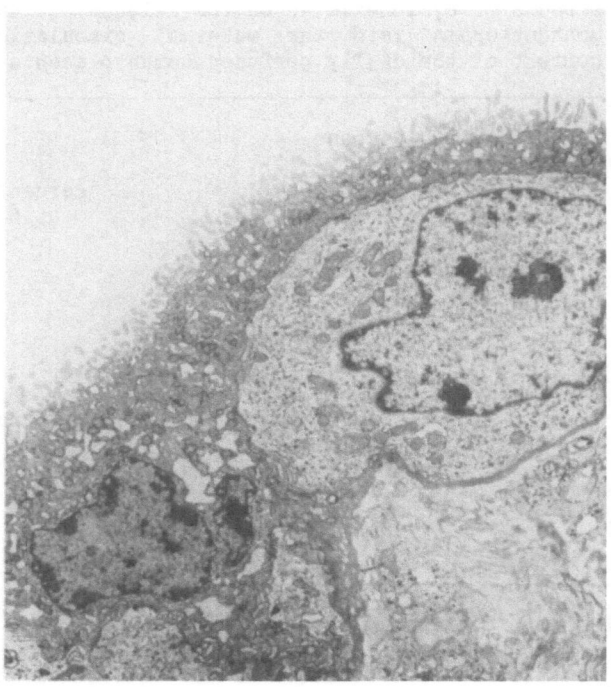

Figure 4.   Twelve-hour perfused placental lobule. Normal structure
compared to preperfused control specimens (x 6700).[40]

TOXICITY SCREENING

Among the most important reasons for undertaking extended perfusions is
to detect the effect of xenobiotics on placental function. In some
instances, immediate effects of an agent on the placenta may be seen;
however, for other substances a longer time may be required at what would
be considered in utero exposure doses – for example, cycloheximide effect
on hCG release and tissue content (Table III). Thus, large concentrations
added initially with a response within minutes or seconds may not reflect
what normally would be happening in utero at lower doses.

For toxicity screening the usefulness of the *in vitro* dually perfused
human placental preparation is that the concentrations can be based on the
known pharmacokinetics in humans or animals. Quite often it is possible to
mimic the blood curves for a particular compound. With such dosing regimens
and perfusions in excess of 12 hours it becomes possible to assess
biochemical alterations, such as enzyme induction or DNA adduct formation.
An example of this possibility is cadmium, a heavy metal, which is often
considered to be a nephrotoxin. In rodents cadmium has been found to
produce fetal death and placental necrosis within 16 hours following a
single subcutaneous dose, and direct placental toxic effects within six
hours.[46-50] Peak maternal blood levels of cadmium were 20 nmoles/ml within
approximately five minutes of administration.[51]

Studies involving human placental perfusions over 12 hours resulted in
a dose related production of lesions, including necrosis of the placenta,
as well as induction of fetal leak. Production and release of human
placental lactogen and human chorionic gonadotrophin were reduced within 5-

6 hrs, as was zinc transfer to the fetal circuit. Interestingly, co-administration of zinc can protect against some of these toxic responses to cadmium.[49] Thus, a similar pharmacokinetic pattern as in the rodent - as well as time sequence and dose response - could be achieved *in vitro* for the human placenta.

This example of cadmium demonstrates that the human placental perfusion model when extended for periods of 12 hours can be used to examine not only the movement and metabolism of substances, but also toxic responses which may take hours to produce *in vivo*. Such capabilities allow better comparisons between animal models and the human.

It is hoped that the challenge of extended perfusions of the human placental lobule will be accepted, and the model further developed to investigate placental pathology and the effects of drugs and toxins, as well as for basic physiological and biochemical investigations.

Acknowledgements

The authors are grateful for the technical assistance of Jeanette Zavislin, Lynn Neth, and Karen DeMesy-Jensen and wish to thank the physicians and nursing staff at the Strong Memorial and Highland Hospitals in Rochester, New York. The research discussed in this contribution was supported in part by grants from the National Institutes of Health (ES 02774 and ES 01247).

REFERENCES

1. Cédard, L. (1973) Placental perfusion *in vitro*. *Acta Endocrinol.* Suppl. **69**, 158, 331.
2. Zrubek, H., Grudzien, M., Sawulicka-Oleszczuk, H., Oleszczuk, J., Panczyk, T. and Czajka, R. (1985) Influence of fenoterol on glucose utilization by the human placenta in an *in vitro* perfusion system. *Contrib. Gynecol. Obstet.* **13**, 168.
3. Krantz, K.E. and Panos, T.C. (1959) Apparatus for establishment of separate extracorporeal fetal and maternal circulation in the human placenta. *Am. J. Dis. Child.* **98**, 674.
4. Krantz, K.E., Panos, T.C. and Evans, J. (1962) Physiology of maternal-fetal relationship through extracorporeal circulation of the human placenta. *Am. J. Obstet. Gynecol.* **83**, 1214-1228.
5. Krantz, K.E., Facog, J.B., Yoshida, K. and Romito, J.A. (1971) Demonstration of viability of perfused human term placenta. *Obstet. Gynecol.* **37**, 183.
6. Szabo, A.J., Grimaldi, R.D. and Jung, W.F. (1969) Palmitate transport across perfused human placenta. *Metabolism* **18**, 406.
7. Nesbitt, R.E.L., Rice, P.A., Rourke, J.E., Torresi, V.F. and Souchay, A.M. (1970) *In vitro* perfusion studies of the human placenta, a newly designed apparatus for extracorporeal perfusion achieving dual closed circulation. *Gynecol. Invest.* **1**, 185.
8. Nesbitt, R.E.L., Rice, P.A. and Rourke, J.E. (1973) *In vitro* perfusion studies of the human placenta. *Gynecol. Invest.* **4**, 243.
9. Hamrin, C.E., Conger, W.L., Lindstrom, R.N., Shier, R.W. and Dilts, P.V. jun. (1971) Placental perfusion device. *Am. J. Obstet. Gynecol.* **110**, 422.
10. Maulik, D., Contractor, S.F., Lippes, J. and Knight, A. (1981) Extracorporeal perfusion of the whole human placenta - a new model. *Placenta* Suppl. **3**, 353.
11. Rice, P.A., Nesbitt, R.E.L., Cuenca, V.G., Zhang, W., Gordon, G.B. and Kim, T.J. (1986) The effect of ethanol on the production of lactate,

triglycerides, phospholipids, and free fatty acids in the perfused human placenta. *Am. J. Obstet. Gynecol.* 155, 207.

12. Panigel, M. (1962) Placental perfusion experiments. *Am. J. Obstet. Gynecol.* 84, 1664.

13. Schneider, H., Panigel, M. and Dancis, J. (1972) Transfer across the perfused human placenta of antipyrine, sodium and leucine. *Am. J. Obstet. Gynecol.* 126, 822.

14. Penfold, P., Drury, L., Simmonds, R.J. and Hytten, F.E. (1981) Studies of a single placental cotyledon *in vitro*: I. The preparation and its viability. *Placenta* 2, 149.

15. Illsley, N.P., Penfold, P., Bardsley, S.E., Tracey, B.M. and Aarnoudse, J.G. (1983) The effects of anoxia on human placental metabolism and fetal substrate profiles investigated by an *in vitro* placental perfusion technique. *Trophoblast Research.* 1, 55.

16. Schneider, H. and Huch, A. (1985) Dual *in vitro* perfusion of an isolated lobe of human placenta: Method and instrumentation. *Contrib. Gynecol. Obstet.* 13, 40.

17. Dancis, J., Ghosh, N.K., Jansen, V., Schneider, H., Fallon, R.J. and Cox, R.P. (1979) Secretory proteins in the perfused human placenta. *Biol. Neonate* 35, 188.

18. Schneider, H., Challier, J-C. and Dancis, J. (1981) Transfer and metabolism of glucose and lactate in the human placenta studied by a perfusion system *in vitro. Placenta* Suppl. 2, 129.

19. Penfold, P., Illsley, N.P., Purkiss, P. and Jennings, P. (1983) Human placental amino acid transfer and metabolism in oxygenated and anoxic conditions. *Trophoblast Research.* 1, 27.

20. Challier, J-C., Schneider, H. and Dancis, J. (1972) *In vitro* perfusion of human placenta V. Oxygen consumption. *Am. J. Obstet. Gynecol.* 126, 261-265.

21. Levitz, M., Jansen, V. and Dancis, J. (1978) The transfer and metabolism of corticosteroids in the perfused human placenta. *Am. J. Obstet. Gynecol.* 132, 363.

22. Contractor, S.F. and Stannard, P.J. (1983) The use of AIB transport to assess the suitability of a system of human placental perfusion for drug transport studies. *Placenta* 4, 19.

23. Contractor, S.F., Eaton, B.M., Firth, J.A. and Bauman, K.F. (1984) A comparison of the affects of different perfusion regimes on the structure of the isolated human placental lobule. *Cell Tissue Res.* 237, 609.

24. Brandes, J., Tavoloni, N., Potter, B.J., Sarkzi, L., Shepard, M.D. and Berk, P.D (1983) A new recycling technique for human placental cotyledon perfusion: Application to studies of the fetomaternal transfer of glucose, insulin, and antipyrine. *Am. J. Obstet. Gynecol.* 146, 800.

25. Alsat, E., Duncan, S.L.B. and Beaconsfield, R. (1982) Full term placental perfusion studies. In: "Placenta - The Largest Human Biopsy". Editors: R. Beaconsfield and G. Birdwood, Pergamon Press, pp 91-112.

26. Miller, R.K., Wier, P.J., Maulik, D. and di Sant'Agnese, P.A. (1985) Human placenta *in vitro*: characterisation during 12 hours of dual perfusion. *Contrib. Gynecol. Obstet.* 13, 77.

27. Wier, P.J. and Miller, R.K. (1985) Oxygen transfer as an indicator of perfusion variability in the isolated human placental lobule. *Contrib. Gynecol. Obstet.* 13, 127.

28. Shah, Y. and Miller, R.K. (1985) The pharmacokinetics of phenytoin in the perfused human placenta. *Pediatr. Pharmacol.* 5, 165.

29. Miller, R.K., Mattison, D.R., Panigel, M., Ceckler, T. and Bryant, R. (1987) Kinetics assessment of manganese using magnetic resonance imaging (MRI) in the dually perfused human placenta *in vitro. Environ. Hlth. Persp.* 74, 81-91.

30. Kuhn, D., Crawford, M., Gordon, G. and Stuart, M. (1988) Aspects of *in*

vitro placental perfusion: Effects of hyperoxia and phenol red. *Placenta*. 9, 201.

31. Miller, R.K., Wier, P.J., Shah, Y. and Perez D'Gregorio, R. (1989) Human placental protein production *in vitro*: > 12 hour perfusions. In: "Placental and Endometrial Proteins: Basic and Clinical Aspects." Editors: Y. Tomoda, S. Mizutani, O. Narita and A. Klopper, VSP Utrecht, The Netherlands, pp 453-460.

32. Schneider, H. and Dancis, J. (1987) *In vitro* perfusion of human placenta - A Workshop Report. *Trophoblast Research*. 2, 597-605.

33. Dencker, L., Miller, R.K., Gasiewicz, T. and Rucci, G. (1987) The pharmacokinetics of dioxin (TCDD) in the perfused human placenta. *Teratology* 35, 74A.

34. Challier, J-C. (1985) Criteria for evaluations of perfusion experiments and presentation of results. *Contrib. Gynecol. Obstet.* 13, 32-39.

35. Malek, A., Miller, R.K., Mattison, M., Ceckler, T., Bryant, R., Panigel, M. and Neth, L. (1989) Continual assessment of energy charge in the perfused human placenta using magnetic resonance imaging spectroscopy of phosphorus. *11th Rochester Trophoblast Conference*. In press.

36. Panigel, M. (1971) Morphological evaluation of perfused tissues. *Acta Endocrinol*. Suppl. 158, 74.

37. Panigel, M. (1974) Relation of the ultrastructure of the placenta to its function. In: "The Placenta, Biological and Clinical Aspects". Editors: K.S. Moghissi and E.S.E. Hafex, Thomas, Springfield, Illinois, p 5.

38. Illsley, N.P., Fox, H., Van der Veen, L., Chawner, L. and Penfold, P. (1985) Human placental ultrastructure after *in vitro* dual perfusion. *Placenta* 6, 23.

39. Kaufmann, P. (1985) Influence of ischemia and artificial perfusion on placental ultrastructure and morphometry. *Contrib. Gynecol. Invest.* 13, 18.

40. di Sant'Agnese, P.A., Demesy-Jensen, K., Miller, R.K., Wier, P.J. and Maulik, D. (1987) Long term human placental lobule perfusion - an ultrastructural study. *Trophoblast Research* 2, 549.

41. di Sant'Agnese, P.A. and Demesy-Jensen, K.L. (1984a) Dibasic staining of large epoxy tissue sections and applications to surgical pathology. *Am. J. Clin. Pathol.* 81, 25.

42. di Sant'Agnese, P.A. and Demesy-Jensen, K.L. (1984b) Diagnostic electron microscopy on re-embedded "popped off" areas of large spur epoxy sections. *Ultrastruct. Pathol.* 6, 247.

43. Perez-D'Gregorio, R., Miller, R.K. and Wier, P.J. (1985) Vitamin B_{12}: transport and metabolism in the *in vitro* perfused human placenta. *10th Rochester Trophoblast Conference*, p 39.

44. Perez-D'Gregorio, R. and Miller, R.K. (1986) Preferential release in endogenous cyanocobalaminin the perfused human placenta. *Placenta* 7, 447.

45. Amstey, M., Miller, R.K., Menegus, M.A. and di Sant'Agnese, P.A. (1988) Non-polio enterovirus infection in pregnant women and the perfused placenta. *Am. J. Obstet. Gynecol.* 158, 775-782.

46. Parizek, J. (1964) Vascular changes at sites of oestrogen biosynthesis produced by parenteral injection of cadmium salts: The destruction of the placenta by cadmium salts. *J. Reprod. Fertil.* 7, 263.

47. Levin, A.A., Plautz, J.R., di Sant'Agnese, P.A. and Miller, R.K. (1981) Cadmium: placental mechanisms of fetal toxicity. *Placenta* Suppl. 3, 303-318.

48. Levin, A.A., Miller, R.K. and di Sant'Agnese, P.A. (1983) Heavy metal alterations of placental function. In: "Development and Reproductive Toxicity of Metals". Editors: T. Clarkson, G. Nordberg and P. Sager, Plenum Press, New York, pp 663-654.

49. Shah, Y., Neth, Y.L., Perez D'Gregorio, R. and Miller, R.K. (1989) Cadmium toxicity in the human placenta *in vitro*: Effect of zinc. *11th Rochester Trophoblast Conference*. In press.

50. di Sant'Agnese, P.A., Jensen, K., Levin, A.A. and Miller, R.K. (1983) Placental toxicity of cadmium: an ultrastructural study. *Placenta* **4**, 149–163.

51. Levin, A.A., Kilpper, R. and Miller, R.K. (1987) The pharmacokinetics of a fetal toxic dose of cadmium chloride administered subcutaneously to the pregnant rat. *Teratology* **36**, 163–170.

EVALUATION OF AN *IN VITRO* DUAL PERFUSION SYSTEM FOR THE STUDY OF PLACENTAL PROTEINS: ENERGY METABOLISM

H. Schneider,[1] A. Malek,[1] R. Duft,[1] and N. Bersinger[2]

Universities of Berne[1] and Zurich,[2] Switzerland

The *in vitro* perfusion of human placenta offers several attractions to the investigator of placental function. Species differences which must be considered when data from animal experiments are discussed are of no concern and there are no ethical or safety questions. Furthermore the isolated *in vitro* situation allows the controlled modification of various experimental conditions. As in other *in vitro* techniques - for example, slices or membrane preparations - the tissue function is being studied after isolation from its natural environment, so considerable differences from *in vivo* behaviour are likely. Maternal and fetal influences which affect placental function by continuously modifying the "perfusate" are excluded, which is advantageous but at the same time present limitations in the interpretation of data.

There is a long-standing tradition of using *in vitro* perfusion systems to study the endocrinology of the human placenta, and extensive data on steroid metabolism were accumulated by Cédard and co-workers a number of years ago.[1] Simultaneous perfusion of the fetal and maternal compartments of an isolated cotyledon of the placenta by two separate perfusion circuits[2] has found widespread acceptance to investigate a broad spectrum of functional aspects of the human placenta.[3] Separate perfusion of the intervillous space has improved the metabolic functions of the tissue and this has been particularly important for the study of placental proteins, since all proteins synthesised by the trophoblast which have been studied so far are released in large amounts into the maternal perfusion stream while only traces are detectable in the fetal compartment.

The functional integrity and the degree of disturbance of the physiological condition must be critically evaluated in interpretation of the results and the limitations of the technique appreciated. We report here recent studies on aspects of placental energy metabolism, which are at the basis of various energy-dependent functions of the placenta. In addition, some data on the integrity of the membrane barrier separating maternal and fetal compartment and its dependence on energy metabolism are presented.

STUDY OF TISSUE METABOLITES

Tissue samples were taken immediately after obtaining the placenta from 32 vaginal deliveries and 16 Caesarean sections. All deliveries occurred at term after normal pregnancies and all newborn infants were in good condition at birth. Tissue samples were taken from the maternal side of the placenta midway between the centre and the periphery of the organ and were freeze-clamped in liquid nitrogen using special clamping forceps.

For analyses of the metabolites the frozen tissue was pulverised to a fine powder at the temperature of liquid nitrogen and 6 grammes of tissue powder were mixed with 15 ml of ice-cold 0.6 M perchloric acid for deproteinisation. The mixture was homogenised in a Polytron tissue homogeniser for one minute. The suspension was centrifuged at 4500 r/min for 30 minutes. Standard enzymatic methods based on the NAD/NADH principle were used to measure the following acid-soluble tissue metabolites in the supernatant of the homogenate: lactate, ATP and creatine phosphate.[4] The spectrophotometric measurements were performed on a Beckman DU-8 spectrophotometer.

Nine placentae, five from vaginal deliveries and four from Caesarean sections, were kept in a bath of physiological saline at 4°C, and tissue samples were taken every five minutes up to 50 minutes to study the change in tissue concentration of various metabolites as a function of time after cord clamping.

PERFUSION STUDIES

Fourteen term placentae, obtained after normal deliveries and uneventful pregnancies, were used for perfusion experiments. The dual *in vitro* perfusion of an isolated cotyledon was performed as described in detail elsewhere.[5] After cannulation of a paired chorionic artery and vein the corresponding villous capillary system was rinsed free of blood. When the isolated lobule had been fixed in a perfusion chamber five metal cannulae were introduced into the intervillous space through the decidual plate and connected to a second perfusion circuit for perfusion of the maternal compartment. The perfusions were performed under controlled conditions with respect to temperature, perfusion pressure, and flow in both circuits. After 15-20 minutes of open system perfusion in both circuits recirculation of a fixed volume of 110 ml each was started on the fetal and maternal side.

Earle's buffered electrolyte solution diluted with tissue culture medium (1:2) was used as perfusing fluid with the following additions: 70 000 Dextran 10 g/l, human serum albumin 4 g%, Clamoxyl 1 g/l, and heparin 10 000 U/l. Radioactive glucose (0.6 µCi D-(U-^{14}C)-glucose) was added to the maternal and fetal circuits and for studies of the permeability of the placental membrane antipyrine (8 mg/100 ml) and creatinine (15 mg/100 ml) were added to the maternal side only. Samples were taken separately from the fetal and maternal circuits at the beginning of perfusion and after 15, 30, 45, 60, 90 and 120 minutes and the same volume of the original perfusate replaced in each circuit. At the end of perfusion the perfused tissue was excised and weighed and tissue samples frozen in liquid nitrogen.

In four of the 14 experiments blood was added to the perfusate using leucocyte-free fresh blood (less than 24 hours old). Fresh blood was mixed with Earle's culture medium in proportions of 100 ml blood to 300 ml medium, and 60 ml of human serum albumin (20%) as well as 250 mg Clamoxyl and 4 000 U heparin were added. Since there is some release of potassium due to haemolysis, a potassium-free buffer was used for dilution. The diluted blood solution had a mean haematocrit and haemoglobin of 16.67 ± 1.15% and 8.03 ± 2.39 g% respectively.

The 14 perfusion experiments were subdivided into three groups with respect to oxygenation. In group 1 the perfusate was equilibrated with a gas mixture of 95% oxygen and 5% CO_2, while in group 2 a 95% N_2 and 5% CO_2 mixture was used in both circuits. The blood-containing perfusate was oxygenated using a membrane oxygenator[6] with a gas mixture containing 20% O_2, 5% CO_2 and the rest N_2. Oxygenation was not entirely satisfactory since mean arterial PO_2 was 88 ± 9.6 mmHg and saturation of haemoglobin was 95.57 ± 4.61%.

Analyses

Antipyrine was measured colorimetrically[7] using a Technicon automated analyser which was also used to perform the enzymatic determination for glucose and lactate. Creatinine was measured by an enzymatic method.[8] Radioactivity was counted after adding 15 ml scintillant (Instagel, Packard Instruments) to 1 ml sample volume in a liquid scintillation spectrometer (Beckman LS-1801) with automatic quench correction using appropriate standards. Total radioactivity was separated into neutral and charged compounds by using ion exchange column chromatography.[9] Acid metabolites were separated from neutral compounds with Dowex 1 x 8 resin as formates and elution was performed with 2N formic acid. An acidified sample (pH 1.0) was put on Dowex 50 W x 8 to bind compounds with a positive charge such as amino acids and subsequently eluted with 2N NH_4OH.

Statistical comparisons were made using the U-test from Mann and Whitney. All mean values are given ± s.d.

RESULTS

Tissue Metabolites

Tissue concentration of lactate was significantly higher while ATP was lower in placentae from vaginal deliveries compared with Caesarean section placentae (Table I). Creatine phosphate concentrations were very low and showed no significant difference between the two groups. The mean time interval between cord clamping, sampling, and freezing of placental tissue was approximately twice as long for placentae from vaginal deliveries.

Table I Tissue levels of ATP, creatine phosphate and lactate in fresh human placentae (Mean ± SD)

	ATP (μmol/g wet wt)	Creatine Phosphate (nmol/g wet wt)	Lactate (μmol/g wet wt)	Time Lag (min)
Caesarean sections	0.453+0.153 n = 16	48.67+29.16 n = 6	3.37+2.13 n = 16	7.5+2.5 n = 16
Vaginal deliveries	0.348+0.151 n = 32	37.00+22.20 n = 5	6.77+2.50 n = 32	16.0+6.5 n = 32
	p < 0.05	n.s.	p < 0.001	p < 0.001

Tissue was freeze clamped in liquid nitrogen. Time lag extends from cord clamping till sampling.

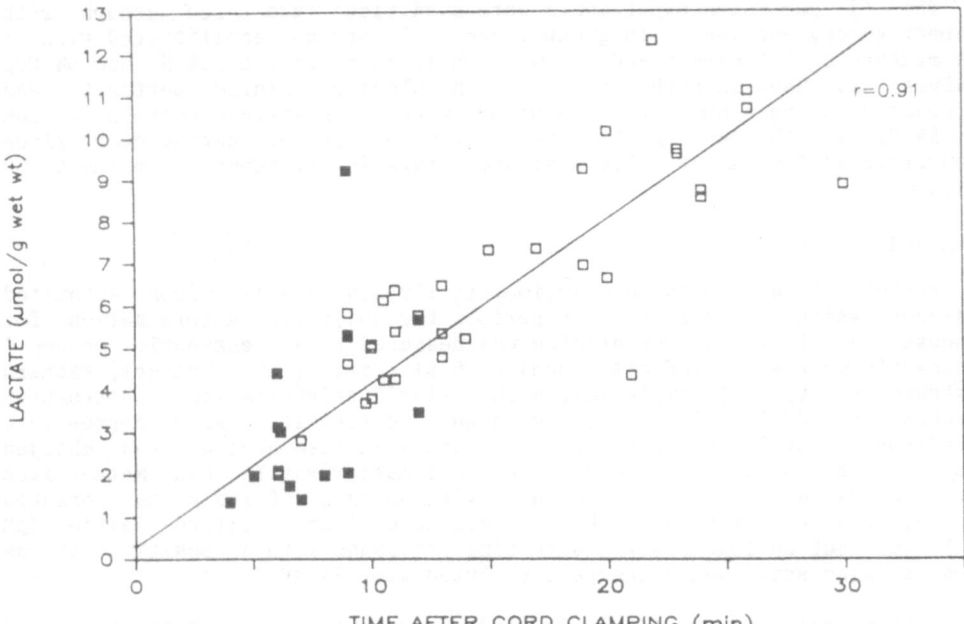

Figure 1.   Influence of ischaemia on placental lactate concentration after clamping of the umbilical cord. □ = Placenta
from Caesarean sections; ■ Placentae from vaginal
deliveries.

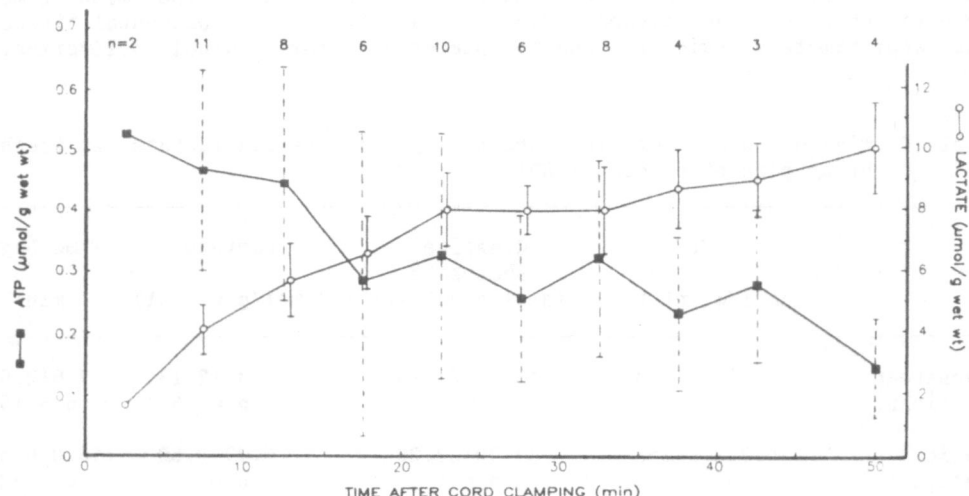

Figure   2.   Change in placental lactate and ATP concentration
following delivery.   Mean values ± SD from nine
placentae (4 CS, 5 VD) which were kept in a bath of
physiological saline at 4°C.

There was a close correlation between tissue lactate levels and time interval between cord clamping and tissue samples (Fig. 1). The difference in tissue metabolites between the placentae from vaginal deliveries and Caesarean sections can be explained by the delay in taking samples after vaginal delivery. From the rise in tissue lactate with increasing time interval between cord clamping and sampling a mean lactate production of 0.350 µmoles/g/min can be calculated, which is similar to the production of lactate observed during oxygenated perfusion.[10] When placental tissue was cooled to 4°C in a bath of physiological saline the initial rise in tissue lactate concentration was similar to that seen under conditions of warm ischaemia, but with cooling of the tissue the curve for lactate flattened earlier and there was less accumulation within the tissue (Fig. 2).

Perfusion Studies

During the two hours of recirculation there was a continuous decline in glucose concentration and a rise in lactate. There was no difference in these changes between fetal and maternal compartments (Fig. 3). From the concentration changes, the perfusate volumes in the two circuits, and the weight of the perfused tissue mean rates of glucose consumption of 6.96 ± 2.50 and lactate production of 21.23 ± 7.79 µmol/h/g were calculated for the experiments with buffer perfusate and 95% oxygen (Table II). In the experiments with 95% nitrogen complete anoxia was not achieved because of some gas permeability of the tubing in the circuit. Arterial PO_2 values were 33.56 ± 17 mmHg indicating that oxygen supply to the tissue was considerably reduced. Under these conditions glucose consumption almost doubled and was significantly higher than in the series with 95% oxygen, while lactate production rose only slightly. In the experiments with diluted blood, glucose consumption was also significantly higher – but lactate production was lower – although the difference did not reach statistical significance.

The overall production of lactate was high, and when converted into glucose equivalents (one mole glucose is equivalent to two moles of lactate) it is apparent that in the experiments with 95% O_2 there is more production of lactate than consumption of glucose (Table III). By separation of radioactive counts on ion exchange columns and the use of specific radioactivity the amount of glucose which is converted into lactate can be calculated. In the experiments with 95% oxygen 77% of

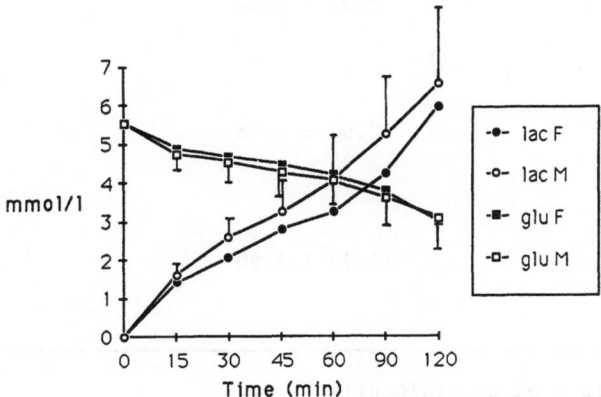

Figure 3. Glucose consumption and lactate production during *in vitro* perfusion with recycling of maternal and fetal circulation with buffer equilibrated with 95% O_2 and 5% CO_2.

Table II   Consumption of glucose and production of lactate during dual *in vitro* perfusion of a human placental cotyledon (Mean ± SD)

Oxygenation	Glucose consumption	Lactate production
	$\mu mol/h/g$	
95% O_2 + 5% CO_2 n = 5	6.96 ± 2.50	21.23 ± 7.79
95% N_2 + 5% CO_2 n = 5	12.50 ± 3.36[1]	24.06 ± 5.24
Air + 5% CO_2 Blood, n = 4	13.75 ± 3.90[2]	15.69 ± 6.69

[1] and [2] compared to 95% O_2 + 5% CO_2: [1] $p < 0.05$, [2] $p < 0.02$

Glucose consumption and lactate production derived from enzymatic determination.

Table III   Production of lactate in percent of glucose consumption

Oxygenation	Glucose consumption $\mu mol/h/g$	Lactate in %
95% O_2 + 5% CO_2 n = 5	6.96 ± 2.50	153
95% N_2 + 5% CO_2 n = 5	12.50 ± 3.36	100[1]
Air + 5% CO_2 Blood, n = 4	13.75 ± 3.90	57[2]

[1] compared to air + 5% CO_2 (blood): $p < 0.05$
[2] compared to 95% O_2 + 5% CO_2: $p < 0.05$

Lactate production was converted into glucose equivalents by dividing it with a factor 2 and then expressed in percent of glucose consumption.

glucose was metabolised to lactate, while with diluted blood only 22% of glucose consumption can be accounted for by production of lactate (Table IV).

We did not specifically measure oxygen consumption in this series of experiments, but on the basis of previous studies[11] we would expect a considerable increase in oxygen consumption with diluted blood as perfusate. It therefore would seem reasonable that a higher percentage of glucose would have been metabolised to CO_2. Since the system was not airtight attempts to recover $^{14}CO_2$ failed and we cannot provide data on overall CO_2 production. We have however calculated the overall recovery of radioactivity including the counts found in tissue extract and surprisingly there was no significant difference between the three groups. The mean recovery was 85.5 ± 8.5%. With a substantially higher fraction of aerobic glycolysis in the blood experiments we would have anticipated a lower recovery in these experiments. Rather unexpectedly we found that up to 50% of the radioactivity in the perfusate at the end of the experiment was precipitable with perchloric acid, indicating that in these experiments substantial amounts of glucose were channelled into protein metabolism.

When the amount of lactate derived from glucose is compared with total lactate production it is seen that a substantial fraction is derived from other sources. This fraction is 49%, 32%, and 62% for the perfusions with 95% oxygen, 95% nitrogen, and diluted blood respectively.

The major portion of the radioactivity recovered by acid extraction from the tissue was identified as lactate, with only slight differences among the three groups (Table V).

Table IV   Production of lactate in percent of glucose consumption

Oxygenation	Glucose consumption µmol/h/g	Lactate in %
95% O_2 + 5% CO_2 n = 5	6.96 ± 2.50	77
95% N_2 + 5% CO_2 n = 5	12.50 ± 3.36	65[1]
Air + 5% CO_2 Blood, n = 4	13.75 ± 3.90	22[2]

[1] compared to air + 5% CO_2 (blood): $p < 0.05$
[2] compared to 95% O_2 + 5% CO_2: $p < 0.05$

Lactate production was derived from specific radioactivity after separation of ^{14}C-lactate and ^{14}C-D-glucose by column chromatography and converted into glucose equivalents for calculation of percent glucose conversion to lactate.

Table V   Tissue radioactivity (Mean ± SD)

Oxygenation	Glucose	%	Lactate
95% O_2 + 5% CO_2 n = 5	23.23 ± 5.64		76.93 ± 6.01
95% N_2 + 5% CO_2 n = 5	16.73 ± 5.70		87.25 ± 7.05
Air + 5% CO_2 Blood, n = 4	35.95 ± 14.73		70.70 ± 13.41

Glucose and lactate are expressed in % of total radioactivity extracted from the tissue.

STUDY OF PERMEABILITY OF THE PLACENTAL MEMBRANE

The permeability was studied using two inert compounds – antipyrine, which is highly lipid-soluble and diffuses rapidly across membranes, and creatinine which has a low degree of lipid-solubility so that there is considerable resistance to its diffusion across membranes. Both compounds were added to the maternal side and due to the concentration difference diffusion occurs into the fetal compartment. When the concentration measured in the fetal perfusate is expressed in percent of the concentration found at the same time in the maternal compartment, after 15 minutes antipyrine reaches 75% of the maternal concentration and after 30 minutes is over 90% and equilibration between the two circuits is almost complete. In contrast after 15 minutes creatinine is at 25% only and even after two hours there remains a significant difference in concentration between fetal and maternal compartments with the concentration in the fetal compartment approximately 70% of that in the maternal concentration. There was no difference in diffusion for these two compounds in the three experimental groups and the mean values for all 14 experiments are shown in Figure 4.

While different conditions of oxygenation with resultant differences in glucose metabolism apparently have little effect on membrane permeability for antipyrine and creatinine, a dramatic change in membrane integrity was seen when glycolysis is suppressed with iodoacetate. In two experiments 0.2 mM iodoacetic acid was added after one hour of perfusion (oxygenation with 95% O_2), and while glucose consumption and lactate production during the first hour were similar to the mean values found in the control group, under iodoacetic acid glucose consumption was reduced by 12% and lactate production by 55%. In four additional experiments 0.2 mM iodoacetic acid was added from the very beginning and there was a drastic reduction in both glucose consumption (67%) and lactate production (88%). The suppression of glycolysis was also demonstrated in the tissue extract with more than 90% of radioactivity recovered as glucose. There was an increasing leak with fluid shift from the fetal to the maternal compartment, indicating

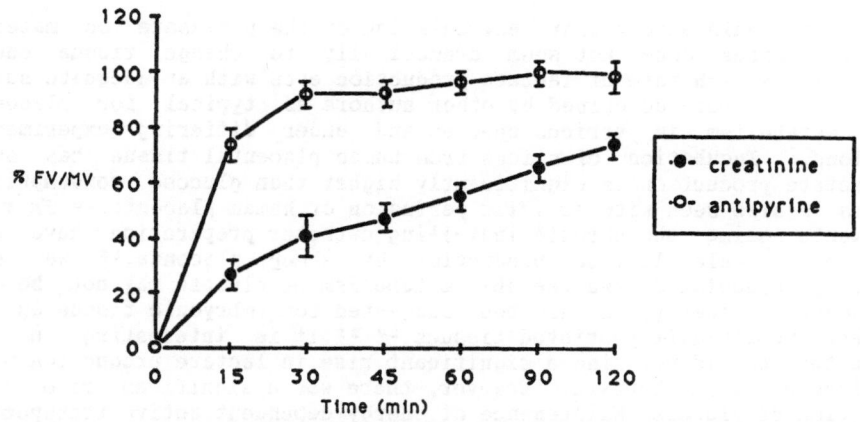

Figure 4.   Concentration of antipyrine and creatinine in the fetal
circulation expressed in percent of maternal   concentration.

deterioration of membrane function.   Normally there is very little bulk
flow of perfusate in spite of a hydrostatic pressure gradient from the
fetal to the maternal side.   After addition of iodoacetic acid there was a
rapidly increasing shift of fluid and the experiments had to be terminated
after 60 minutes.   A similar rise in bulk flow was also observed with 2,4-
dinitrophenol.[12]

DISCUSSION

One of the disadvantages of *in vitro* perfusion of the freshly delivered
human placenta is a variable period of partial or total ischaemia which
begins with the clamping of the umbilical cord.   The perfusionist has only
limited control over the length of time before *in vitro* perfusion of fetal
and maternal compartments can be started.   The extent of tissue changes
induced by ischaemia may influence the result of perfusion experiments and
further tissue changes may develop with reperfusion because of the toxic
effect of oxygen introduced into ischaemic tissue. The rise of lactate seen
with increasing time intervals between cord clamping and tissue sampling
permits the calculation of mean lactate production, which is similar to
previously determined values under conditions of dual *in vitro* perfusion.[10]
Therefore it seems there is no increased lactate production as a result of
accelerated glycolysis during ischaemia, which is in agreement with our
findings on lactate production during perfusion under conditions of anoxia
or hypoxia.   The tissue concentrations measured immediately after delivery
for ATP or lactate are similar to those reported by other investigators[13]
as was the further rise in tissue lactate with the placenta maintained at
4°C.   A rapid initial drop in tissue ATP occurs during the first minute of
ischaemia as shown in the guinea-pig placenta as well as in the human
placenta.[14,15]   It seems however that after the initial rapid drop further
loss of ATP is less rapid, and a constant level is maintained at around
0.2-0.3 ATP µmol/g. With start of perfusion it was possible to bring tissue
ATP levels back to the immediate post-delivery value of around 0.5
µmol/g.[12] In general, due to the specifics of tissue metabolism, there may
be a higher resistance to ischaemia in fetal and placental tissues by
better preservation of tissue ATP compared with adult tissues.[16]

The total of glucose consumption and lactate production using 95%
oxygen and 5% CO_2 is similar to our results using perfusion of both
circuits in open circuit.[10]

Thus it would appear that recirculation of the perfusate on maternal and fetal sides does not seem dramatically to change tissue energy metabolism. A high rate of lactate production even with an adequate supply of oxygen has been described by other authors as typical for placental tissue metabolism in various species and under differing experimental conditions. Incubation of slices from human placental tissue has shown that lactate production is significantly higher than glucose consumption[17] and this is also seen with *in vitro* perfusion of human placenta.[18] *In vivo* experiments using the chronic indwelling catheter preparation have also shown considerable lactate production by sheep placenta.[19] We have previously speculated that aerobic metabolism of glucose may not be the prime source of energy, as has been suggested for embryonic tissue as well as other poorly-differentiated tissues.[20,21] It is interesting in this context that we did not find a significant rise in lactate production under conditions of tissue hypoxia. However, there was a significant rise in the consumption of glucose. Maintenance of energy-dependent active transport of amino acids under conditions of severe tissue hypoxia using the *in vitro* perfusion of human placenta has been observed.[22]

For a more detailed description of glucose metabolism the use of labelled glucose as a tracer is required. There is but little information on studies using radioactive glucose in human placental tissue. Incubation of placental slices showed that 69% of the tracer was metabolised to lactate and 1.6% to CO_2.[23] This was recently confirmed, with conversion of 80% of labelled glucose into lactate and only 2% to CO_2.[24] With labelled glucose in the perfusion system only 10.4% of the tracer extracted from the perfusate – and not recovered on the fetal side – was found as lactate and 3.4% as CO_2; more than 85% of the radioactive glucose was unaccounted for.[25] The experimental conditions were not entirely comparable, since open circuit perfusion was used on the fetal and maternal sides and the radioactive label was added to the maternal side only. We found, in the buffer experiments at least, that the bulk of glucose consumption can be accounted for by lactate production. There was no significant difference in the experiments with 95% oxygen versus anoxia with respect to the percentage of glucose metabolised to lactate. On the other hand total glucose consumption doubled with blood as perfusate; however, the percentage of glucose converted to lactate dropped to only 22%.

Since we could not measure CO_2 production it is not certain whether aerobic glycolysis was substantially increased in the blood experiments. High rates of overall recovery for radioactivity make a large production of CO_2 unlikely, and there was some indication that, using blood, placental protein metabolism was stimulated, and some of the radioactive material became incorporated into proteins.

When the amount of lactate derived from glucose metabolism is compared with total production of lactate, it is clear that there must be additional sources of lactate, and this proportion is considerably higher in the blood experiments (62%) than in the two buffer groups.

It appears that a number of questions about oxidative metabolism in the human placenta have yet to be answered.

Acknowledgements

We wish to thank Barbara Benz for expert technical assistance. This work was supported by funds from the Schweizerische Nationalfonds.

48

REFERENCES

1. Cédard, L. (1971) Placental perfusion *in vitro*. In: "Perfusion techniques". Editor: E. Diczfalusy. 4th Karolinska Symposium, pp 331-346, New York.
2. Panigel, M. (1969) Placental perfusion. In: "Fetal homeostasis". Editor: R. Wynn. Vol. 4. Appleton Century Crofts, p 15, New York.
3. Schneider, H. and Dancis, J. (1985) *In vitro* perfusion of human placental tissue. International Workshop, Zurich 1984, Karger, Basel.
4. Bergmeyer, H.V. (1974) Methods of enzymatic analysis. 2nd Edition, Weinheim: Verlag Chemie, New York: Academic Press.
5. Schneider, H. and Huch, A. (1985) Dual *in vitro* perfusion of an isolated lobe of human placenta: Method and instrumentation. In: "*In vitro* perfusion of human placental tissue". Editors: H. Schneider and J. Dancis. S. Karger, Basel.
6. Folkman, J., Cole, P. and Zimmerman, S. (1966) Tumour behaviour in isolated perfused organs *in vitro*, growth and metastases of biopsy material in rabbit thyroid and canine intestinal segment. *Ann. Surg.* **164**, 491.
7. Brodie, B.B., Axelbrod, J., Soberman, R. and Levi, B.B. (1949) The estimation of antipyrine in biological materials. *J. Biol. Chem.* **179**, 25-29.
8. Heinegard, D. and Tiderstrom, G. (1973) Determination of serum creatinine by a direct colorimetric method. *Clin. Chim. Acta.* **43**, 305.
9. Kreisberg, R.A., Siegal, A.N. and Owen, W.C. (1972) Allanine und gluconeogenesis in men: Effect of ethanol. *J. Clin. Endocrinol.* **34**, 876-883.
10. Soda, R.J., Proegler, M. and Schneider, H. (1984) Transfer and metabolism of norepinephrine studied from maternal to fetal and fetal to maternal sides in the *in vitro* perfused human placental lobe. *Am. J. Obstet. Gynecol.* **148**, 474-481.
11. Challier, J.C., Schneider, H. and Dancis, J. (1976) *In vitro* perfusion of human placenta. V. Oxygen consumption. *Am. J. Obstet. Gynecol.* **126**, 261-265.
12. Bersinger, N.A., Malek, A., Benz, B., Keller, P.J. and Schneider, H. (1988) Effect of protein synthesis inhibitors and metabolic blockers on the production of placental proteins by the *in vitro* perfused human placenta. *Gynecol. Obstet. Invest.* **25**, 145-151.
13. Carroll, M.J. and Young M. (1987) Observations on the energy and redox state on protein synthetic rate in animal and human placentas. *J. Perinat. Med.* **15**, 21-30.
14. Carroll, M.J. and Young M. (1982) Mixed protein synthetic rate in the tissue of the isolated lobule of the human placenta. *J. Physiol.* **332**, 5.
15. Bloxam, D.C. and Bobinski, P.M. (1984) Energy metabolism and glycolysis in the human placenta during ischaemia and in normal labour. *Placenta* **5**, 381-394.
16. Harkness, R.A., Coade, S.B., Simmonds, R.J. and Duffy, S. (1985) Effect of a failure of energy supply on adenine nucleotide breakdown in placentae and other fetal tissues from rat and guinea pig. *Placenta* **6**, 199-216.
17. Holzmann, J.R., Philipp, A.F. and Battaglia, F.C. (1979) Glucose metabolism, lactate and ammonia production by the human placenta *in vitro*. *Pediatr. Res.* **13**, 17.
18. Schneider, H., Challier, J.C. and Dancis, J. (1981) Transfer and metabolism of glucose and lactate in the human placenta studied by a perfusion system *in vitro*. *Placenta* (Suppl 2.), 129-138.
19. Burd, L.J., Jones, M.D., Simmons, M.A., Makowski, E.L., Meschia, G. and Battaglia, F.C. (1975) Placental production and fetal utilization of lactate and pyruvate. *Nature* **254**, 710-711.
20. Warburg, O. (1925) The metabolism of carcinoma cells. *Am. J. Canc.* **IX**, 148-163.

21. Sweeney, M.J., Ashmore, J., Morris, H.P. and Weber, G. (1963) Comparative biochemistry of hepatomas. IV. Isotope studies of glucose and fructose metabolism in liver tumours of different growth rates. *Canc. Res.* 23, 995-1002.
22. Penfold, P., Illsley, N.P., Purkiss, P. and Jennings, P. (1984) Human placental amino acid transfer and metabolism in oxygenated and anoxic conditions. *Trophobl. Res.* 1, 27-36.
23. Sakuray, T., Takagi, H. and Hosoya, N. (1969) Metabolic pathways of glucose in human placenta: Changes with gestation and with added 17-estradiol. *Am. J. Obstet. Gynecol.* 105, 1044-1054.
24. Lopez-Bernal, A. (1984) Corticosteroid metabolism by human intra-uterine tissues in relation to parturition. D. Phil. Thesis, University of Oxford.
25. Challier, J.C., Hauguel, S. and Desmaizières, V. (1985) Metabolism and transfer of radioactive glucose in the human placenta studied by dual perfusion. *Contrib. Gynec. Obstet.* 13, 144-146.

DE NOVO SYNTHESIS OF PREGNANCY-SPECIFIC AND PREGNANCY-ASSOCIATED PROTEINS

BY THE *IN VITRO* PERFUSED HUMAN TERM PLACENTA

Niklaus A. Bersinger,[1] A. Malek[2] and H. Schneider[2]

Universities of Zurich[1] and Berne[2], Switzerland

Placental perfusion is one of several *in vitro* techniques to investigate the production of pregnancy proteins by the trophoblast as well as their control mechanisms. The preparation as described in the chapter by Schneider et al is a closed-circuit system – that is, the released proteins and hormones accumulate in the circulating perfusate. This has the advantage of consuming less medium and yielding smaller volumes of more concentrated solutions when compared with the open perfusion protocol. We are aware that the release kinetics may differ between open and closed circuit protocols. For this reason we have abandoned our first protocol which required a full medium change after two hours of perfusion[1] and have followed a new one which required the removal of 5 ml aliquots from both circuits every 30 minutes during the first two hours and every 60 minutes thereafter. The removed aliquots were replaced with fresh medium injected into both circulations.

PERFUSION IN PRESENCE AND ABSENCE OF METABOLIC INHIBITORS

Despite the lack of knowledge about their biological function pregnancy proteins can be tentatively grouped into three main categories.[2] Group one consists of exclusively trophoblastic proteins – for example hCG, hPL, and SP$_1$. They cannot be detected outside pregnancy. Group two proteins are also mainly of trophoblastic origin during pregnancy but are produced by non-trophoblastic tissues as well. PAPP-A, the most prominent member of this category, has been found to be synthesised by endometrial cells in culture.[3] The last group consists of maternally produced proteins which are present in non-pregnancy sera but show a substantial increase during gestation; α_2-Pregnancy Associated Glycoprotein (α_2-PAG) is an example.

The perfusion system described was used to obtain information on the placental synthesis and release of pregnancy proteins in the absence of maternal tissue. The lobule was prepared and the experiments carried out as described in the preceding chapter by Schneider and colleagues. The medium was 33% Earle's supplemented with mixed amino acids (6.3 mg/ml), human serum albumin (40 mg/ml), Dextran 40 000 (10 mg/ml), Clamoxyl (0.5 mg/ml) and various nutrients. A portion (2–4 g) of unperfused placental tissue adjacent to the lobule selected for perfusion was freeze-clamped in liquid nitrogen; the same was done with the perfused lobule itself at the end of the experiment. These tissue samples were later extracted with isotonic buffer. Four major fractions were obtained from each experiment:

M = maternal perfusate at the end of the experiment
F = fetal perfusate at the end of the experiment
B = extract of unperfused tissue (taken as "tissue extract before per-
    fusion")
A = tissue extract of the perfused lobule after the experiment.

In addition the aliquots removed from the two circuits at regular time
intervals (as explained) were available. The perfusing medium itself was
used as control in all determinations.

In the first analysis only the tissue extracts before and after
perfusion (B and A) were taken into account. PAPP-A, hCG, hPL, SP₁, and
α₂-PAG were determined either by RIA or ELISA using commercially available
kits or methods developed in our laboratory. The values were normalised for
the wet weight of the lobule and expressed per gramme of tissue. Prolactin
was determined with an in-house RIA and haemoglobin with the cyanmethaemo-
globin technique. This latter protein was used as a control non-placental
marker and the results were processed as above. For each individual
pregnancy protein the ratio AFTER:BEFORE perfusion (A:B) was calculated.
The results are presented in Figure 1. Haemoglobin, prolactin and α₂-PAG
showed A:B ratios below 0.22; they were removed from the tissue during
perfusion. The group including hCG, hPL, SP₁, and PAPP-A had ratios of 0.62
or above. The highest A:B values were obtained for hPL.

This clear distinction of the trophoblastic proteins from the others is
an indication of synthesis but might also be the consequence of a slower
release. However, we have shown that de novo synthesis occurred (see
below).

During closed perfusion the concentrations of the above proteins in the
circulating medium increased with time, the fetal concentration remaining
less than 5% of the maternal level.[1] This fetal:maternal concentration

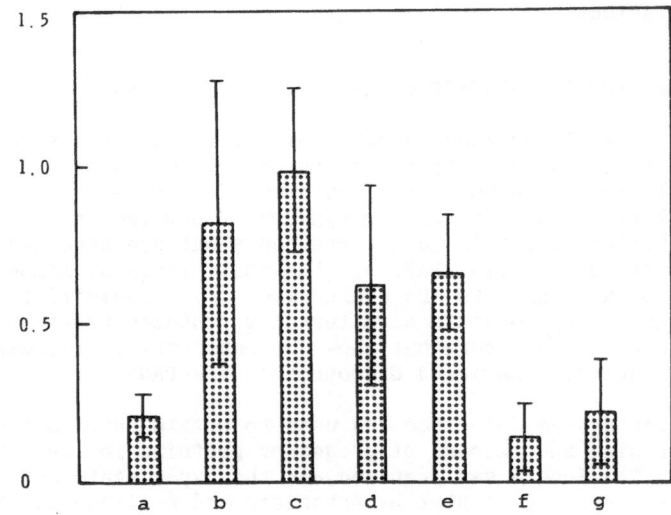

Figure 1.   Specific protein content in unperfused (A) and perfused
            (B) tissue. The bars show the ratio A:B as means and
            standard deviations; n = 5. a = haemoglobin; b = hCG; c
            = hPL; d = SP₁; e = PAPP-A; f = α₂-PAG; g = Prolactin.
            Reprinted from[4] with permission by S. Karger Ltd.,
            Basle.

ratio was found to increase with perfusion time and to be inversely proportional to the molecular weight of the protein, suggesting a slow, passive leak through the membrane barrier from the maternal into the fetal compartment. Such increases in concentration over time in the maternal perfusate were also observed for α_2-PAG and haemoglobin, presumably due to washout of serum from the intervillous space.

NET SPECIFIC SYNTHESIS (NSS)

In order to distinguish fresh biosynthesis from the release of preformed protein it was necessary to calculate the total amounts of each protein in each of the four major fractions (M, F, A, B) present at the end of the experiment. This was done using the following formulae:

$$M_{TOT} = [M] \times V_M \times f_M$$

$$F_{TOT} = [F] \times V_F \times f_F$$

where V were the perfusate volumes and f the correcting factors accounting for the removals and replacements of medium during the course of the perfusion. For example, in a run with five removals/replacements of 5 ml each time and a constant no-leak volume of 120 ml perfusate we could find:

$$f = (120/115)^5 = 1.24.$$

Knowing the amounts of analyte present in the placental extracts per gramme of tissue (from the calculation of the A:B ratios presented in Fig. 1) and the weight W of the perfused lobule (20 - 50 g), the NSS can be calculated, using

$$NSS = A + \frac{M_{TOT} + F_{TOT}}{W} - B.$$

The results obtained over five perfusion experiments are shown in Table I. For each protein hCG, hPL, SP$_1$, and PAPP-A not only the NSS itself but also the ratio NSS:B is tabulated. This ratio relates the quantity of material produced to the tissue extracts before perfusion. This reflects the *in vivo* situation (amount present in serum) to some extent. This mode of calculation also obviates the need for units and enables us to compare one placental protein to another. The values clearly show that hPL was produced to a greater extent than the other proteins; but the range was wide (1.98 to 12.8). This hPL dominance can be explained on one hand by the fact that the peak production of this hormone *in vivo* takes place in the third trimester (the opposite of hCG) and, on the other hand, by the comparatively small molecular weight and higher release rate per unit time.[4] However, yet another unknown mechanism controlling hPL production under *in vitro* perfusion conditions cannot be excluded.

PERFUSION IN PRESENCE OF SYNTHESIS INHIBITORS AND UNCOUPLERS

The effect of protein synthesis inhibitors and metabolic blockers on the production of placental proteins was investigated in order to strengthen the evidence for de novo synthesis during *in vitro* perfusion.[4] The perfusion time is short when compared to tissue culture experiments involving such inhibitors. For this reason we decided to use the inhibitors at the following final concentrations: (i) cycloheximide, 100 µg/ml; (ii)

Table I. Net Specific Synthesis (NSS) and NSS : B ratios (see text) for four placental proteins. All values are means ± SD (n = 5)

	NSS	NSS : B
hCG	40.2 ± 32.3 IU/g	1.38 ± 0.89
hPL	211. ± 68.2 μg/g	6.21 ± 4.39
SP₁	41.2 ± 11.9 μg/g	0.93 ± 0.24
PAPP-A	61.3 ± 35.5 mIU/g	2.17 ± 1.21

puromycin, 10 μg/ml; (iii) iodoacetic acid, 0.2 mM; and (iv) 2,4-dinitrophenol (DNP), 1 mM. They were added after 30 minutes of closed perfusion to both maternal and fetal circulations. Three placentae were perfused with each inhibitor (four with DNP). The perfusions were run for three hours or until a dramatic fluid leak from the fetal to the maternal circulation prevented continuation. This was the case with iodoacetic acid and with DNP where the leakage developed 15 to 20 minutes after the addition of the blocker and where the perfusion had to be stopped after 75–105 (iodoacetic acid) or 90-120 minutes (DNP), respectively. With cyclohex-imide or puromycin no such leakage was observed.

Allowing for the shorter perfusion intervals for iodoacetic acid and DNP we calculated the NSS as explained earlier. The results are presented graphically in Figure 2.

The strongest inhibiting effect was observed with iodoacetic acid, in spite of the short perfusion period. With this blocker the NSS of all four analysed proteins was strongly and significantly reduced. This is not surprising since iodoacetic acid interferes early in glycolysis, thus blocking not only the respiratory chain but also the lactate pathway which remains open in the presence of DNP. However, even DNP was efficient in reducing the NSS of the proteins tested, indicating that the placenta still makes considerable use of oxidative phosphorylation. The protein synthesis inhibitors interfering at the translational level (cycloheximide, puromy-cin) also decreased the NSS of the proteins tested, but this effect was not always statistically significant. Only hPL was clearly affected by all four inhibitors which confirms the data presented in Figure 1.

These results provide evidence that mainly hPL, but also hCG, SP₁, and PAPP-A are produced by the placenta in the absence of maternal tissue during *in vitro* perfusion.

PERFUSION IN PRESENCE OF LABELLED AMINO ACIDS

Direct evidence of synthesis can be obtained through the incorporation of labelled amino acids into protein during perfusion. The situation, however, is not very favourable for this type of experiment because the total time of perfusion is short when compared to cell or organ culture experiments. The stores of ready activated amino acids at the beginning of the perfusion might be sufficiently large to prevent the incorporation of freshly produced labelled aminoacyl-tRNA. In order to meet these problems we decided to use a comparatively high dose of labelled precursors and to omit the cold amino acids in the medium altogether.

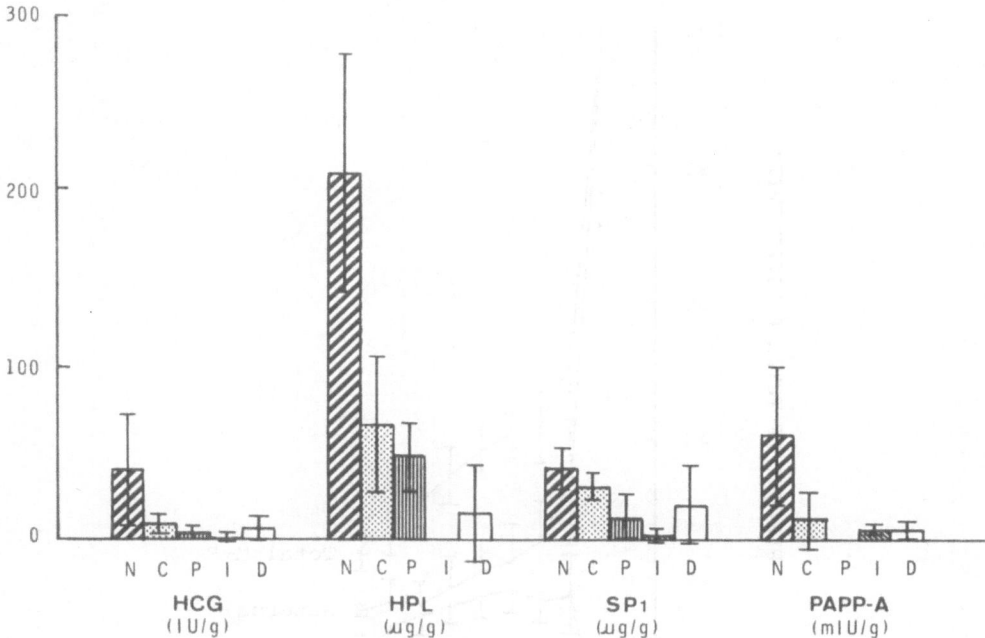

Figure 2. Net Specific Synthesis (NSS) of pregnancy proteins during *in vitro* perfusion, in absence (N) and presence of cycloheximide (C), puromycin (P), iodoacetic acid (I), or 2,4-dinitrophenol (D). The bars are means ± SD. For explanations and calculations see text. Reprinted from[4] with permission by S. Karger Ltd. Basle.

After a short control interval (15-20 min) of closed perfusion the tracer (125 µCi of ^{14}C-L-Amino Acid mixture from New England Nuclear, Cat. No. NEC-445E) was added to the medium of the maternal circulation. This moment was considered t = 0. From then on, the perfusion experiment was continued with the regular removal of medium as described above. No other drugs (inhibitors, etc.) were added in this series of perfusions (n = 7). The aliquots withdrawn at t = 120 minutes and thereafter were not replaced with fresh medium to prevent excess dilution. The perfusion was run as long as possible - that is, as long as the fluid leak from the fetal to the maternal compartment was below 10 ml. In the last three experiments of this type (runs 32, 33, 34) a perfusion time of six hours (from the addition of the tracer) was achieved.

Distribution of Radioactivity

The concentration of label in the maternal and fetal circulation is shown in Figure 3 as a function of time (mean and SD of runs 27-33). Similar concentrations of total tracer in both circuits were reached after 30-90 minutes of perfusion (the difference between the two was not significant over all six experiments when taken together). The total circulating radioactivity (sum of M and F, corrected for the volume) decreased significantly with perfusion time and, after six hours, made up less than 40% of the initial radioactivity.

The isotonic tissue extract A (using three to four volumes of buffer) contained another 13 - 35% of the label, resulting in a total yield of 55.8% ± 7.5 (SD) % (n = 7). To investigate the fate of the remaining 45% of

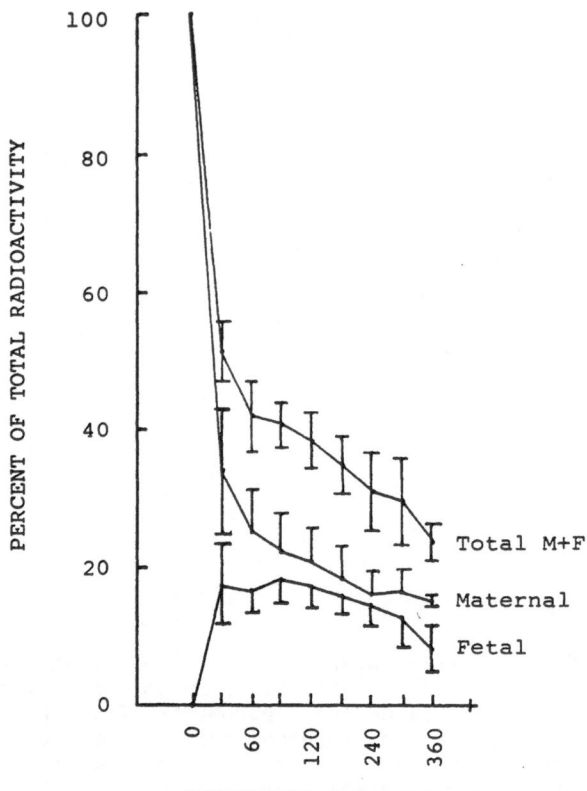

Figure 3. Concentration of circulating radioactivity in the maternal and the fetal circulation as a function of time.

the counts, the post-perfusion tissue pellet of experiment no. 44 obtained after homogenisation and centrifugation was further extracted with the same isotonic buffer ("Wash"), then with 1.5 M NaCl ("High Salt") followed by 2% (v/v) Triton X-100 ("Triton Extract") in TBS. With this method another 7.4% in total of the label could be recovered (Table III). One third of the counts, however, was unextractable by mild techniques. The stepwise extraction protocol is now being improved, but in spite of these efforts a considerable amount of label is lost - that is, it binds strongly to the insoluble fraction of the tissue. It is also possible that part of the counts have been lost as $^{14}CO_2$ through metabolism of the labelled amino acids by oxidative phosphorylation.

Incorporation of Labelled Amino Acids into Protein

The fraction of protein-bound radioactivity was determined by precipitation in duplicate assays with trichloroacetic acid (TCA). One hundred microlitres (with a known number of counts) of sample (perfusate M or extract A) were first diluted with 150 µl PBS containing human serum albumin 40 mg/ml (that is, the same concentration as in the perfusing medium). Then 500 µl TCA (1 M) were added and the tubes vortexed. After short centrifugation 500 µl of the supernatant were removed and counted. The fraction of precipitated DPM was obtained by differential calculation.

Table II. TCA precipitation of perfusates and tissue extracts. The figures are given in percent of the total DPM present in the tested aliquot

Run	Maternal Circulation								Fetal	Tissue
No.	30	60	90	120	180	240	300	360	End	End
27	2.0	5.7	6.1	12.1	23.3	24.1	21.5	-	7.0	46.4
29	ND	4.1	ND	9.8	14.7	16.2	17.6	-	0.1	45.2
30	ND	ND	ND	ND	15.7	-	-	-	0.2	43.0
31	ND	ND	ND	ND	4.8	-	-	-	0.1	36.1
32	0.1	2.0	5.9	8.6	7.9	ND	18.7	19.2	1.4	49.0
33	0.1	2.3	7.0	10.1	16.7	19.4	ND	22.0	1.5	41.1
44	ND	2.9	ND	6.5	9.0	11.3	12.1	12.6	5.9	36.8

Maternal circulation - time course in minutes
ND - not determined

Table III. Yield and distribution of label in perfusion 44

	DPM x 10^6		Percent	
Total (Introduced)	264.1		100.0	
Maternal perfusate	48.2		18.3	
protein-bound		6.1		12.6
free		42.1		
Fetal perfusate	46.7		17.7	
protein-bound		2.8		5.9
free		43.9		
Isotonic tissue extract	37.8		14.3	
protein-bound		13.9		36.8
free		23.9		
Isotonic tissue wash	6.6		2.5	
protein-bound		2.6		39.4
free		4.0		
High salt extract	3.4		1.3	
protein-bound		2.0		57.9
free		1.4		
Triton extract	9.5		3.6	
protein-bound		6.1		64.4
free		3.4		
Lost	111.9		42.3	
Total protein-bound		33.5		12.7

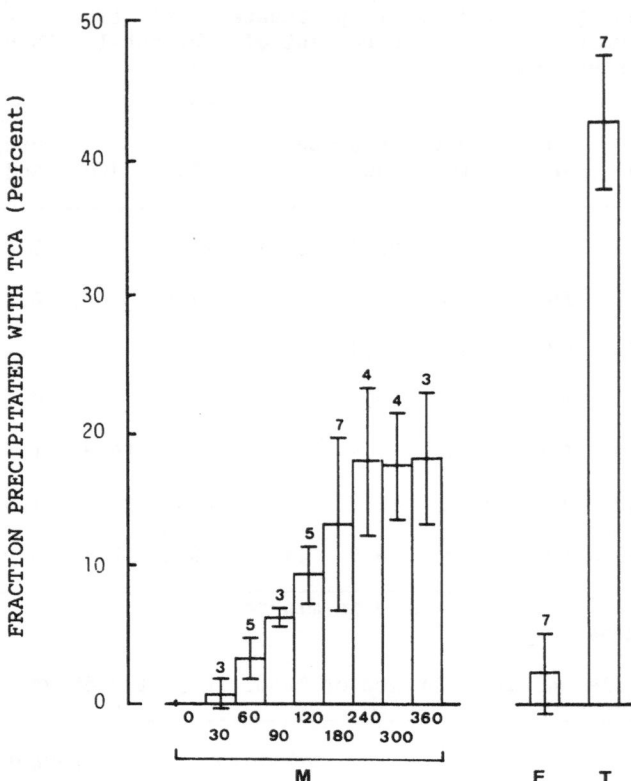

Figure 4.   Fraction of label, in perfusates and extracts, which is precipitated with TCA. M = maternal; F = fetal circulation; T = tissue extract A.   The values for the maternal circulation are shown as a function of time. The bars are means ± SD; the n value is stated on top of the error bar.

Table II and Figure 4 show the mean fraction of protein bound counts in the maternal circulation (as a time course), fetal circulation (at the end) and in the isotonic tissue extract. Protein-bound label increases on the maternal side during the first four hours of perfusion. The plateau which follows can be explained first by the decrease of metabolic (synthetic) activity of the placenta after four hours of perfusion followed by the fluid leak into the maternal compartment, which results in a dilution of the latter with labelled free amino acids since the fraction of protein-bound label on the fetal side is small. The tissue extract, on the other hand, has a high (around 40%) fraction of counts as TCA-precipitable material; one might imagine that the intracellular compartment contains a large element of protein or protein precursors which have been synthesised, and therefore labelled, but have not yet been released.

The yield of free and TCA-bound radioactivity is shown on the pie chart in Figure 5 (experiments 27 - 33). The observation that 14% of the introduced counts are precipitated with TCA after an exposure of six hours or less demonstrates a high synthetic activity. With a total load of 125 µCi this amount corresponds to 17.75 µCi (38.6 x 10^6 DPM) or 318 nmoles amino acid equivalents. The mean weight of the perfused lobule was 32.5 g (range 16 - 49); in other words approximately 10 nmoles of labelled amino acids, per gramme of tissue wet weight, were incorporated into protein.

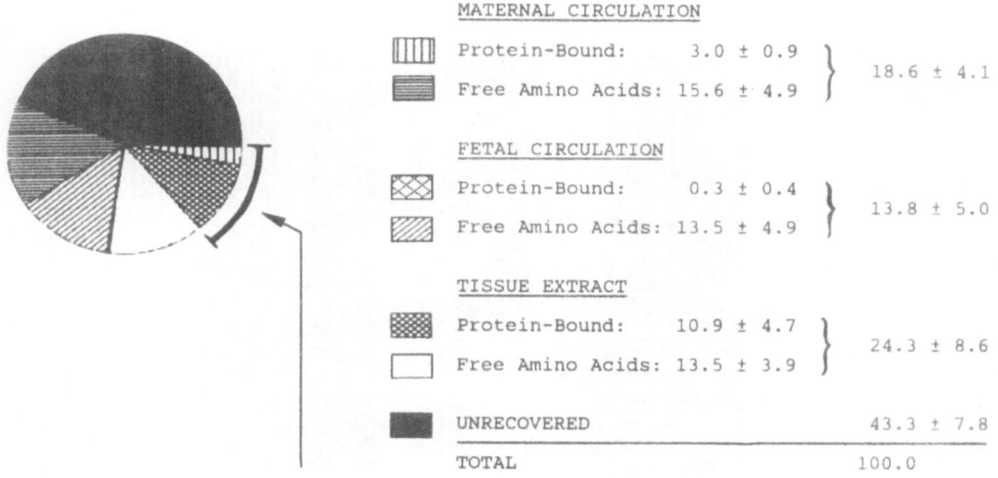

MATERNAL CIRCULATION		
Protein-Bound:	3.0 ± 0.9	} 18.6 ± 4.1
Free Amino Acids:	15.6 ± 4.9	
FETAL CIRCULATION		
Protein-Bound:	0.3 ± 0.4	} 13.8 ± 5.0
Free Amino Acids:	13.5 ± 4.9	
TISSUE EXTRACT		
Protein-Bound:	10.9 ± 4.7	} 24.3 ± 8.6
Free Amino Acids:	13.5 ± 3.9	
UNRECOVERED		43.3 ± 7.8
TOTAL		100.0

TOTAL RECOVERED PROTEIN-BOUND COUNTS: 14.2 % OF INTRODUCED COUNTS

Figure 5.   Distribution of label, after perfusion, between isotonic tissue extract A and the circulations M and F. Each
of these three compartments is divided into protein-
bound (TCA-precipitable) and free radioactivity. The
values are means of 6 perfusions (27 - 33) and SD. Note
that the protein-bound fraction in the fetal perfusate
could not be shown on the pie since it makes up only
0.3% of the total.

The distribution of radioactivity in the various fractions of experiment 44 are analysed in more detail in Table III and illustrated in Figure
6. The overall area of the blocks corresponds to the total amount of label
in a particular fraction, while the level of the light grey portion at the
bottom indicates the percentage of protein-bound label in that fraction.
The Figure shows that, in the tissue extracts, this percentage increases
with further extraction. The labelled protein recovered in the Triton
extract could have been membrane-bound (specifically or non-specifically),
but it cannot be excluded that the previous extraction steps had been
incomplete, leaving soluble intracellular protein behind which is then
released after disruption of the membranes by the detergent.

IMMUNOPRECIPITATION

In order to detect de novo synthesised pregnancy proteins immunoprecipitation with specific antibodies against hCG, hPL, SP1, PAPP-A and α_2-PAG
was performed on maternal perfusates M and tissue extracts A of experiments
32 and 33. Labelled protein was concentrated by dialysis and lyophilisa-
tion. Reconstitution buffer was added to yield 150,000 DPM/ml, approximately. Immunoprecipitation was performed in duplicate with 500 µl sample and
25 µl undiluted antibody (from Dakopatts) or rabbit immunoglobulin. This
amount of antibody was found to be sufficient to bind all antigen present
in the sample. After incubation at 37° C (2 hours) and 4° C (overnight) the
second antibody, donkey anti-rabbit-IgG from the Scottish Antibody Production Unit, was added (375 µl/tube) and the incubation repeated as before.
After centrifugation, the pellets were washed twice with phosphate buffered
saline and counted.

Significant amounts of label were immunoprecipitated by all the
hyperimmune antibodies except by anti-α_2-PAG where the value equalled the

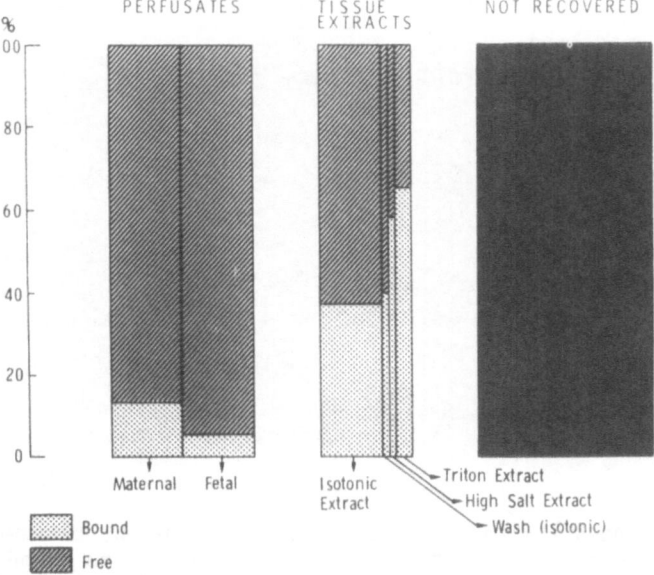

PERFUSATES   TISSUE EXTRACTS   NOT RECOVERED

Maternal   Fetal   Isotonic Extract   → Triton Extract   → High Salt Extract   → Wash (isotonic)

Bound

Free

Figure 6.   Yield and distribution of label in perfusion run no. 44 (see Table III). The principle of this figure is explained in the text. Note that the protein-bound fraction in the fetal perfusate was high when compared with the other control runs (Table II).

Table IV.   Immunoprecipitation of de novo synthesised pregnancy proteins. All values are in nmoles amino acid equivalents and per gramme of perfused tissue

Run 32	Maternal Perfusate	Fetal Perfusate	Tissue Extract	Total
hCG	0.041	0	0.145	0.186
hPL	0.284	0.008	2.077	2.369
SP$_1$	0.314	0.004	1.226	1.314
PAPP-A	0.064	0	0.314	0.378
α_2-PAG	0	0	0.041	0.041
Total Protein	2.18	0.08	12.12	14.38
Run 33	Maternal Perfusate	Fetal Perfusate	Tissue Extract	Total
hCG	0.105	0.001	0.120	0.226
hPL	0.614	0.016	1.031	1.661
SP$_1$	0.253	0.001	0.462	0.716
PAPP-A	0.210	0	0.249	0.459
α_2-PAG	0.082	0	0	0.082
Total Protein	3.46	0.23	7.96	11.65

one obtained with the control non-immune rabbit IgG. This background was much smaller for the maternal perfusates (2.8-3.4% of introduced counts) than for the tissue extracts (18.4-20.4%). After subtraction of the background and conversion into specific radioactivities the results shown in Table IV were obtained. Of our panel of proteins examined, hPL was detected in large quantities confirming the findings presented by Schneider and co-workers elsewhere in this volume. SP$_1$ was next largest in amount after hPL. PAPP-A and hCG production was small but still significant and without difference between perfusates and extracts.

The values obtained for α_2-PAG as well as all figures for fetal perfusates are not significant above background.

CONCLUSIONS

The production of pregnancy proteins by the perfused placenta during a limited but controlled time interval can be demonstrated by two different approaches: effect of metabolic synthesis inhibitors and incorporation of labelled amino acids as precursors. Both showed that of the proteins tested, hPL was the one produced in highest amounts, followed by SP$_1$. These are both specific to the placenta and show, *in vivo,* their highest serum concentrations in the third trimester. The production (and sensitivity to cycloheximide for example) of hCG was less pronounced, probably because term placentae were used and hCG was over its peak of synthesis. PAPP-A, on the other hand, is a high molecular weight entity and its release might be slow though at peak activity at term. These differences between the proteins illustrate their independent behaviour. The mechanisms that control their production and release can be studied with the model described here.

Acknowledgements

We thank Ms. B. Benz, Zurich, and Mss. E. Aegerter and U. Knuchel, Berne, for skilled technical assistance with the perfusions. Part of this work was supported by a grant no. 3.916-85, of the Swiss National Science Foundation.

REFERENCES

1. Bersinger, N.A., Schneider, H. and Keller, P.J. (1986) Synthesis of placental proteins by the human placenta perfused *in vitro* (preliminary report). *Gynecol. Obstet. Invest.* 22, 47 - 51.
2. Chard, T. and Grudzinskas, J.G. (1985) Placental and pregnancy-associated proteins: Control mechanisms and clinical application. In: "Proteins of the Placenta". Editors: P. Bischof and A. Klopper. Karger, Basle, pp 279 - 287.
3. Bischof, P. and Tseng, L. (1986) *In vitro* release of pregnancy-associated plasma protein A (PAPP-A) by human endometrial cells. *Am. J. Reprod. Immunol. Microbiol.* 10, 139 - 142.
4. Bersinger, N.A., Malek, A., Benz, B., Keller, P.J. and Schneider, H. (1988) Effect of protein synthesis inhibitors and metabolic blockers on the production of placental proteins by the *in vitro* perfused human placenta. *Gynecol. Obstet. Invest.* 25, 145 - 151.

IN VITRO MODELS FOR READING AND MANIPULATING TROPHOBLAST SIGNALS

Arnold Klopper and Garry Luke

Royal Infirmary, Aberdeen, Scotland

Endocrine glands need information. They have to receive messages telling them how much of their hormones to produce and when to secrete them. For most endocrine glands the signalling system is well known, at least in outline. Thus gonadotrophin releasing hormone, a peptide of known constitution coming from the hypothalamus, informs the anterior lobe of the pituitary when and how much luteinising hormone to release. The whole system cannot operate unless there is a feedback from the site of action, telling the endocrine gland of the need for its hormone. The one exception appears to be the placenta. So far no feedback signals controlling the production of its many protein secretions, some of which are hormonal in nature, has been defined. A decade ago this curious circumstance led one endocrinologist to propound the despairing thesis that placental proteins have no biological function. There is no feedback signal from the site of action and the production rate of placental proteins is solely related to trophoblast mass and blood flow in the intervillous space.[1] Seven years later he saw no reason to modify his hypothesis.[2]

One way to look for feedback control over the release of placental proteins is to set up *in vitro* preparations of placenta, feed putative control factors into the system, and examine what happens to the release of specific proteins. Somewhat surprisingly, no comprehensive hypothesis has been put forward to challenge the Chard thesis,[2] although suggestions have been made in respect of individual proteins. For example, it has been shown that epidermal growth factor stimulates the release of hCG and hPL in explant cultures,[3] and a similar effect of gonadotrophin-releasing hormone on hCG release has been found.[4] Such external control factors can operate either on the biosynthesis of new hormone within the trophoblast or on the release of preformed material in the cell cytoplasm. It may be that the trophoblast is geared to a steady low level of hormone release determined by the relationship of the cell to the surrounding fluid medium in terms of such factors as the concentration of calcium or hormone in the medium. The placenta is unique among endocrine glands in that the trophoblast is in direct contact with the bloodstream in the intervillous space, whereas other endocrine gland cells are separated from the circulation by a layer of blood vessel endothelium and its basement membrane at least. Compared to interstitial fluid, the intervillous blood changes rapidly and its relationship with the cytoplasm of the trophoblast is more dynamic than that of an ordinary endocrine cell and its surrounding medium. Before *in vitro* models can be used to test putative *in vivo* stimulatory factors, it is essential to obtain accurate information about the effects of the medium itself on the basal release rate. A survey of the literature on *in vitro* placental models suggests that the basal release rate may vary greatly from time to time in the same experiment in controls not subjected to stimulatory agents. Scant attention has been paid to the dynamics of unstimulated protein release from the placenta.

It is our purpose to present some experimental findings on the release of proteins from the trophoblast and to speculate on the factors which might govern the rate of release. We have considered data obtained from three types of *in vitro* preparations.

The first is explant culture of fragments of trophoblast. The material is obtained from surgical termination of pregnancy (six to ten weeks gestation) and the chorionic tissue is separated from decidua by visual inspection before culture.

The second is dual perfusion of a single lobule of a term placenta as described by Abramovich et al.[5] This technique involves the simultaneous independent perfusion of the fetal vasculature in a single placental cotyledon and of the intervillous space of the corresponding lobule.[6]

The third technique is the superfusion of fetal membranes, clamped between two chambers. This is a method adapted by Mulder and de Bakker-Teunissen from a technique of Ussing and Zerahn[7] used in the superfusion of frog skin.

The placental proteins we have measured are: chorionic gonadotrophin (hCG), placental lactogen (hPL), Schwangerschaftprotein 1 (SP_1), and pregnancy-associated plasma protein A (PAPP-A). There is some controversy whether PAPP-A is of purely placental origin, but as it is certainly released by placental preparations and is a much larger molecule than the other proteins it seems of interest to take it into consideration. We have also measured albumin and prolactin; the former because it is a protein present in trophoblastic tissue but not synthesised there, and the latter because it is secreted into the intervillous space by the decidua. We have also measured two steroids synthesised in the trophoblast - oestradiol and progesterone. They are much smaller molecules than the proteins and it is likely that they are released by a different mechanism from that which operates in the case of the proteins.

TIME COURSE OF PLACENTAL PROTEIN RELEASE

There is a common thread which runs through many *in vitro* experiments on the release of proteins from the trophoblast. It is illustrated in Figure 1, taken from the work of Page and colleagues (see pp 15-24). This shows the release into the maternal circuit of four placental proteins from a series of dual perfusions. The proteins in the effluent were measured at 10-minute intervals and the amount released at each time point expressed as a percentage of the total release over 220 minutes. Although this was an open circuit experiment - that is to say, the perfusate was passed through the cotyledon once only - a similar result is obtained if aliquots are taken from a resevoir of perfusate which is being passed through the intervillous space again and again (closed circuit). The data can be represented in many ways: as a percentage of total release, as the total protein released in each time interval or, best of all, as a release rate - that is, the amount released per unit time and weight of tissue. Whichever way it is expressed and whatever the experimental design, one phenomenon can always be discerned: the release is high at first and falls rapidly with time.

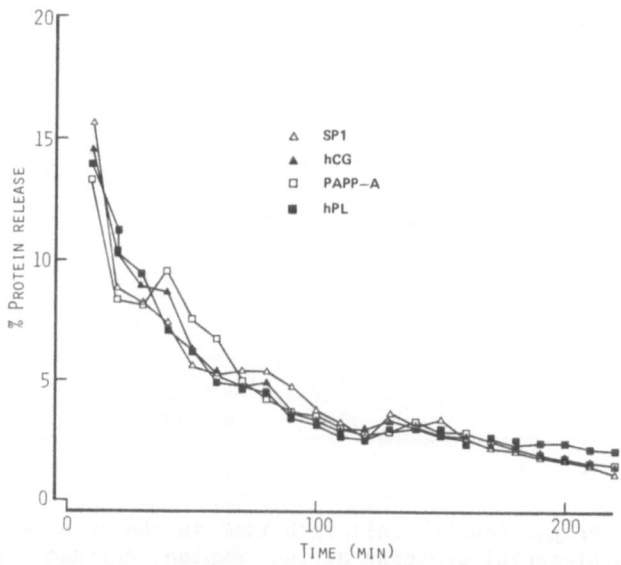

Figure 1. Proportionate fall with time in the release of four
placental proteins during dual perfusion. The points
represent protein release in successive 10-minute periods expressed as a percentage of the total released in
220 min. Each point is the mean from six placentae.

Nor is this a peculiarity of dual perfusion experiments. Figure 2 shows
the same phenomenon observed with placental explants in culture. We were
surprised to find that fetal membranes in dual chamber superfusion also
released placental proteins on both sides, having assumed that this tissue
exercised only barrier, not secretory, functions. Figure 3 once again
demonstrates the pattern of a high initial release followed by a slow
continuous fall in release rate. Although Figure 3 shows only the result
of SP1 assays, similar findings were recorded for hCG, hPL, and PAPP-A. It
is evident that this pattern is not the peculiarity of one particular
model, but represents the behaviour of trophoblast cells under *in vitro*
conditions.

It is difficult to assemble all the findings in real numbers from four
different proteins, as these are released in very different amounts in
different experiments and are measured in different units. Figure 4
presents an idealised representation of the pattern of release. It has not
been extended beyond five hours as we have no figures for dual perfusion or
membrane release beyond this time. The curve is reminiscent of a diffusion
curve, but it may represent a different mechanism. All four of these
proteins are present in the maternal blood, and such a falling curve could
be produced by maternal serum being washed out from the intervillous space
of the perfused cotyledon. However, this explanation could not apply to the
results from membrane release or explant culture. In the case of the
perfused cotyledon, the amount of protein released is far in excess of the
amount which could be contained in the serum remaining in the intervillous
space of a cotyledon, which has an average volume of 5 cc.[8] Clearly, even
in the case of cotyledon perfusion, there is another mechanism operating.
Cell death with consequent leakage of cytoplasmic contents into the medium
has to be considered, but is unlikely. These *in vitro* techniques are well
established and many workers, including ourselves, have adduced evidence of
continuing cell function and the maintenance of normal morphology by
electron microscopy. There may be subtle alterations in membrane permeability, but these have not been noted by physiologists working with *in vitro*

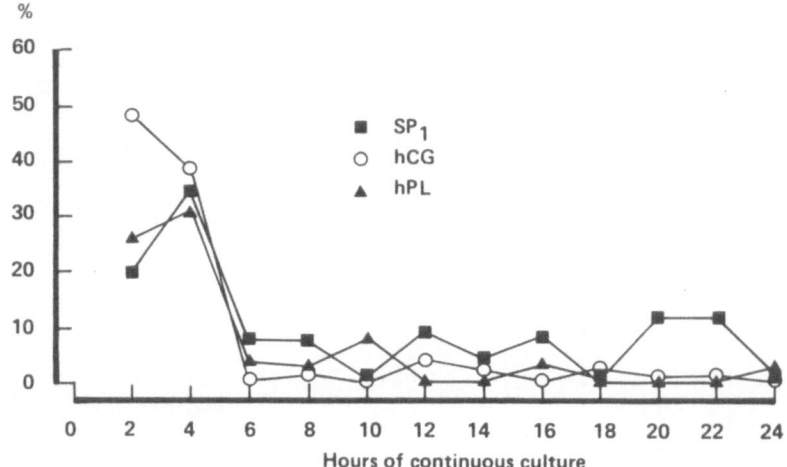

Figure 2. Proportionate fall with time in the release of three placental proteins during explant culture. The points represent the average of six separate cultures from a pool of 10 early placentae.

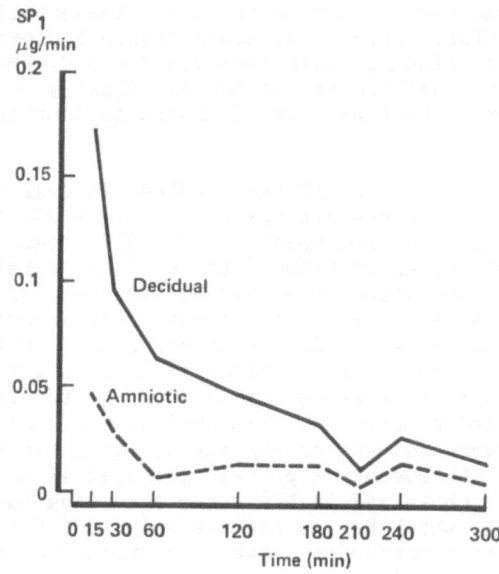

Figure 3. The release rate of SP₁ (μg/min/g) from the decidual and the amniotic face of the placental membranes during superfusion.

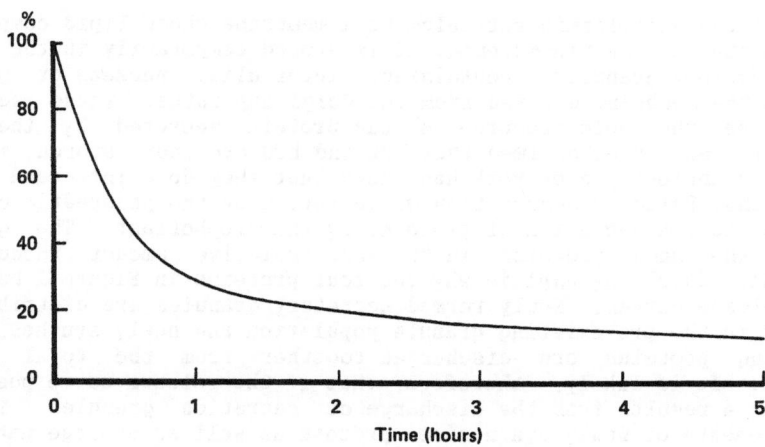

Figure 4.   An idealised representation of the pattern of release
            of placental proteins *in vitro.*

preparations. Biosynthesis of these proteins, for example SP1,[9] is known to
proceed under *in vitro* conditions. It seems likely that the release pattern
is determined by a dynamic interaction between biosynthesis at the level of
the rough endoplasmic reticulum and the subsequent transport of formed
products to the plasmalemma and their discharge through the membrane. It is
a matter of prime importance to the reading and manipulation of trophoblastic signals that the different roles of these mechanisms should be clearly
understood.

     The discharge of formed protein through the cell membrane could be
regarded as analogous to the diffusion of salts through a semipermeable
membrane. Tempting though this idea may be, proteins are not salts and they
pass through cell membranes by exocytosis, not by gradient diffusion.   To
provide one explanation Page has put forward the hypothesis of an unstirred
layer in the intervillous space adjacent to the microvilli of the
syncytiotrophoblast, thus creating a concentration gradient between it and
the flowing medium beyond (see pp 20-21).   While this might well apply to
the intervillous space in perfusion experiments it is difficult to see such
an unstirred layer existing around the cells of an explant in a metabolic
shaker.

     To examine how the discharge of intracellular protein might be coupled
to a gradient diffusion it is necessary to examine more closely how protein
is transported in the cell from its site of synthesis to the plasmalemma
and then through this membrane to the exterior. The model for the
pancreatic cell proposed by Palade[10] may well apply to the trophoblast, at
least so far as intracellular events are concerned. The proteins with which
we are concerned are synthesised by the ribosomes of the endoplasmic
reticulum.   The newly synthesised proteins are segregated in the cisternal
space of the rough endoplasmic reticulum. This segregation from the cell
sol results from changes in the conformation of the proteins - for example,
formation of disulphide bridges or proximal hydroxylation - which make the
protein molecules too large to pass through the cisternal membrane.   They
are then transported to the Golgi apparatus by a system requiring energy,
which is supplied by oxidative phosphorylation. The proteins reach the
condensing vacuoles of the Golgi complex in a dilute solution and are then
greatly concentrated into a secretion granule. If these secretion granules
constitute the starting point of the diffusion gradient just postulated, it
is easy to see why release rates should be high initially. In the Golgi
complex the secretory product is transferred from the high permeability

membrane of the endoplasmic reticulum to a membrane whose lipid composition approaches that of the plasmalemma. It is stored temporarily in the form of mature secretory granules, containing, inter alia, packets of proteins encased in the membrane derived from the Golgi apparatus. These secretory granules are the sole precursor of the proteins secreted by the cell. Although it has been claimed that hPL and hCG are not stored in such secretory granules[11] later work has shown that they do exist[12] and it is apparent that Palade's description of secretion by the pancreatic cell is applicable to the secretion of proteins by the trophoblast. The granules discharge the same proteins in the same relative amount through the plasmalemma, which may explain why the four proteins in Figure 1 have such similar release curves. Newly formed secretory granules are distributed at random within the pre-existing granule population and newly synthesised and pre-existing proteins are discharged together from the total granule population. It is likely, therefore, that if the release curve postulated in Figure 4 results from the discharge of secretion granules, it will contain elements of newly synthesised protein as well as storage material.

If the release curves we have observed represent diffusion gradients the events at the discharge of the granules through the cell membrane are all important, for it is at this point that the gradient will be established. Although highly concentrated, the granules should not be thought of as solid structures. We are talking of the passage of a membrane encased vesicle through the plasmalemma – not of a solid granule. The process of exocytosis is diagrammatically illustrated in Figure 5. It starts with the fusion of the membrane of the granule with that of the plasmalemma. Although this is not shown in Figure 5 several secretory granules may fuse with the one originally adherent to the plasmalemma, thus enlarging the resevoir of concentrated protein which establishes continuity with the outside.[13] Figure 5 shows that the granule vesicle reforms and moves back into the cytoplasm. Palade[10] describes the process thus: "In the case of discharge, the membranes of the secretory granules can be viewed as a set of individual vesicular containers that move forward from the Golgi complex to the surface during exocytosis, and presumably back to the Golgi complex during coupled endocytosis." As will be seen later, endocytosis is important to our hypothesis. It creates the possibility of a protein flux

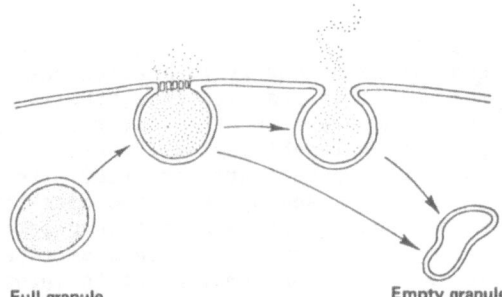

Full granule   Empty granule

Figure 5.   A diagrammatic representation of exocytosis showing two possible mechanisms consonant with the chemical and electron microscopical evidence. Both involve establishing continuity between the contents of the secretory granule and the medium outside the cell, enabling a diffusion gradient to exist. In both instances granule membranes are retained after evacuation of their contents. Reproduced with permission from W.W. Douglas.[13]

across the plasmalemma as presumably the vesicle can carry back into the cell sol proteins which had diffused into it during the time when its contents were in continuity with the outside medium. This fits with the occasional finding of diffuse distribution of hPL and hCG in the cell sol.[11,12]

The process we have described takes no cognisance of specific secretory stimuli which may act either on the biosynthetic, the transport, or the transmembrane passage phases of protein release. The last is also an energy dependent process, one which can be inhibited by colchicine. There are, therefore, specific chemical inhibitors for each step - biosynthesis, transport, and discharge. As discharge can proceed in the absence of continuous synthesis, it is possible to get some impression of the time course of these events by inhibition of specific steps. The time course appears to be different in different cell types; in general biosynthesis is rapid, (a matter of minutes), although transport, particularly the concentration step in the Golgi apparatus, takes three or four hours. If the time course of trophoblast secretion is similar, then the short duration of dual perfusion limits it to reflecting transport and discharge, while changes in culture after three or four hours could be reflecting biosynthetic events.

Much of the design of *in vitro* experiments and the interpretation of the results depend on whether a gradient diffusion between the cell and the surrounding medium is an essential step. Clearly the release rate will depend on the gradient. In dual perfusion under open circuit where proteins do not accumulate in the medium, the gradient is at first steep and the release rate is high. As the number of secretory granules available decreases the release rate drops away to the point where the number of granules discharging are in balance with their replacement by new biosynthesis. It is evident from Figure 1 that this point is not quite reached by the 220 minutes which the experiment lasted. Figure 6, taken from the work

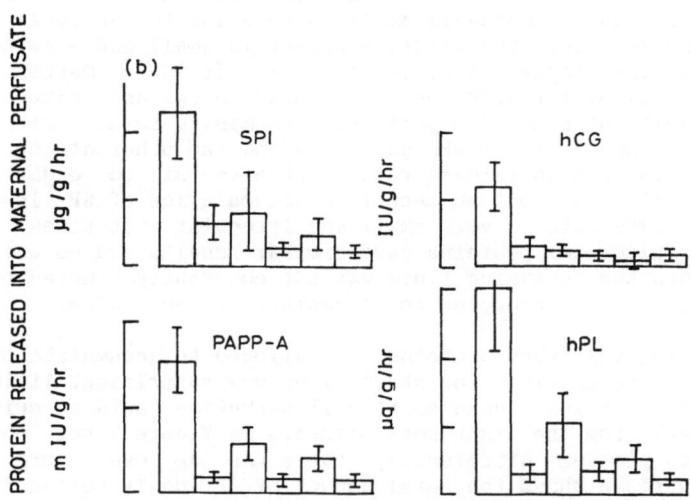

Figure 6.   Release rates of placental proteins during successive
             periods of open and closed circuit. The open circuit
             release rates are shown in the first, third, and fifth
             column of each histogram and the closed circuit results
             in the second, fourth and sixth column. The bars
             represent the SEM of five dual perfusion experiments in
             each case.

of Page and co-workers (see pp 18-19), shows the release rate of four placental proteins during successive periods of open and closed circuit. The release rates, with the exception of some later hCG rates, are always lower under closed circuit than those of both preceding and succeeding periods of open circuit. The distinction between open and closed circuit is very much less sharp with explant culture, as this technique does not involve continuous removal of medium. The gradient then is changing at both ends, becoming less steep as proteins accumulate in the medium and also becoming less steep as intracellular proteins are depleted. There is worse to come: the process is often wholly discontinuous. In many culture experiments the medium is changed at intervals, being wholly replaced by fresh blank medium. This of course tips the gradient back to a steeper slope with its associated higher release rate. It never goes back to the same slope as before because the intracellular protein has been depleted by the previous period of culture. Manoeuvres like pre-incubation merely shift the problem down the line. However, if a particular agent which is presumed to stimulate or inhibit the secretion of a particular placental protein is being tested it is possible to compare test and control cultures over long periods of time, say 24 or 48 hours. But this gives no information about the dynamics of the experiment. It is not known at what time during the culture the test started to deviate from the control. The dynamics of the release rate depends upon the point in the secretion process at which the agent acts. If the effect of colchicine upon the release of SP_1 by the trophoblast in culture were being tested one would expect the release to stop almost immediately, as this agent acts on membrane discharge. On the other hand, cycloheximide, which acts on biosynthesis, may take four or more hours to have a significant effect.

One way to read the dynamics of protein release while still allowing protein to accumulate is to take small aliquots at frequent intervals. Cultures can be kept going for 48 hours or longer enabling the observer to look seriatim at release rates during the phase of release of preformed protein and then later when biosynthetic processes are dominant. The aliquot removed for protein estimation is replaced by blank medium but, provided the volume removed is small in relation to the total volume of medium in the culture, the dilution effect is small and does not greatly tip the gradient toward a faster outflow. It is a matter of simple arithmetic to allow for dilution in calculating release rates. Figure 7 shows the results of such an experiment, examining release rates of SP_1 by two placentae, one at six weeks gestation and the other at ten weeks. At first there is a high release rate, but after six to eight hours the gradient has flattened out so much from accumulation of SP_1 in the medium that the release rate is very small and irregular, at times falling to zero. Other placental proteins gave similar results and so did the fetal membranes when the perfusing fluid was not constantly removed but sampled at intervals, allowing proteins to accumulate in the medium.

The finding that when proteins were allowed to accumulate outside the cells zero release obtained for short times was surprising. It implied that on occasion the complex mechanism of cell secretion could be switched off. When the data from the sixth week placenta in Figure 7 was more closely examined and plotted differently, there was an even more surprising finding. Figure 8 shows the total amount of SP_1 newly released into the medium every two hours. The protein continued to accumulate in the medium for the first 16 hours, rapidly for the first four hours and more slowly thereafter. From 16 to 22 hours, there was no net release; instead the total SP_1 in the medium, allowing for dilution, fell slightly at each time point between 16 and 22 hours. In other words, <u>there is a loss of protein from the medium.</u> These solutions are stable when the tissue is removed from the incubation mixture and it is difficult to conceive of a destructive process which switches on and off when the medium is in contact with the

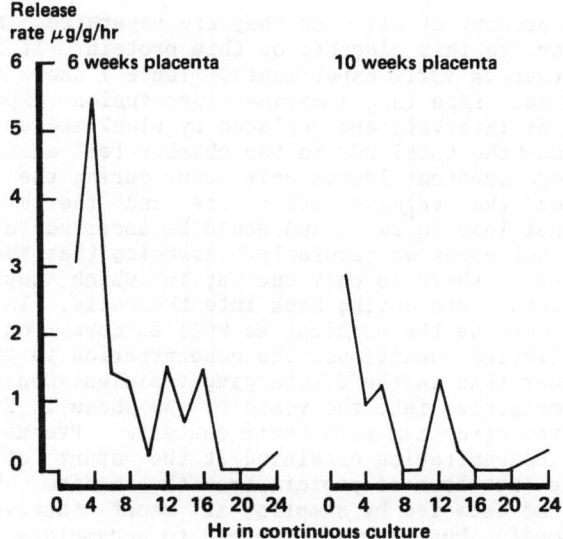

Figure 7. Release of SP₁ in trophoblast cultures with two-hourly sampling.

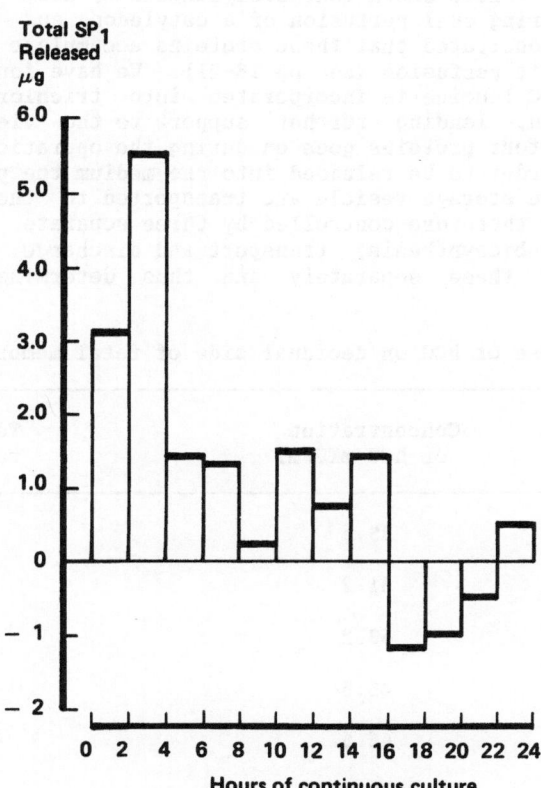

Figure 8. The amount of SP₁ released into the medium at 2 hourly intervals over 24 hours in culture. Positive values indicate the amount by which the total in the medium rose and negative values the amount by which it fell.

tissue and is not present at all when they are separated. Nor is it an aberration, peculiar to this placenta or this protein. It is seen with other proteins in other *in vitro* experiments. Table I shows the release of hCG from the decidual face in a membrane superfusion experiment where aliquots were taken at intervals and replaced by blank medium. This shows that on two occasions the total hCG in the chamber fell during the period of observation. These apparent losses only occur during the latter part of the experiment when the release rate is low and the system is near equilibrium. The net loss is small and could be ascribed to experimental variation if it did not occur so regularly. Assuming that the losses from the medium are real, there is only one way in which they could have occurred: the proteins are moving back into the cells. In a diffusion gradient molecules move up the gradient as well as down - only more move down. At near equilibrium conditions, the concentration in the medium may, on occasion, be higher than in the discharging vesicles. Consequently there will be a flow of molecules into the vesicle. As shown in Figure 5 these vesicles return to the cytoplasm with their contents. Presumably they take back the protein concentration obtaining at the start of endocytosis, accounting for the net loss of protein from the medium. This flux of protein can only be detected by sampling at short intervals, and not removing the whole medium but allowing protein to accumulate.

EFFECT OF BIOSYNTHESIS ON PROTEIN RELEASE

Bersinger et al[14] have shown that biosynthesis of hCG, hPL, SP1 and PAPP-A goes on during dual perfusion of a cotyledon and Page and his colleagues have demonstrated that these proteins accumulate in the tissue during closed circuit perfusion (see pp 18-21). We have found that during explant culture ^{14}C leucine is incorporated into trichloroacetic acid-precipitable protein, lending further support to the view that fresh biosynthesis of all four proteins goes on during the operation of these *in vitro* models. In order to be released into the medium the protein has to be packaged into the storage vesicle and transported to the plasmalemma. The release rate is therefore controlled by three separate (and probably independent) steps; biosynthesis, transport and discharge. It is possible to block each of these separately and thus determine what role

Table I.   Release of hCG on decidual side of fetal membranes

Time min	Concentration of hCG mIU/ml	Total new release mIU
0 - 15	39.5	316
15 - 30	41.2	57
30 - 45	53.2	141
45 - 60	45.5	- 3
60 - 120	46.6	59
120 - 180	50.1	79
180 - 240	41.3	- 15
240 - 300	44.9	91

biosynthesis, transport or discharge is playing at various times in the operation of *in vitro* models. We have looked at the effects of cycloheximide, actinomycin D, and puromycin on the release of proteins in explant cultures. They act at different points in protein biosynthesis. Cycloheximide inhibits transpeptidation, actinomycin binds to DNA and inhibits transcription, while puromycin prevents chain elongation. All three inhibitors have in common inhibition of biosynthesis without affecting the subsequent steps of transport and discharge of the formed protein.

Not surprisingly the results were similar, and for the sake of brevity only the effects of actinomycin will be considered (Tables II and III). At 24 hours all three proteins show a slightly increased concentration with actinomycin compared with controls, possibly because actinomycin causes leakiness of the membranes. By 48 hours the values have moved in the opposite direction and actinomycin-treated cultures now have somewhat lower concentrations than the controls. If it is assumed that actinomycin inhibited biosynthesis without affecting transport or discharge it implies that the 24 hour results are dominated by the high initial release of preformed protein. With this experimental design it is impossible to tell at what point the release of preformed protein ceased to play an important part. Serial sampling, but allowing the protein to accumulate by removing only small aliquots of the total incubation volume, might demonstrate at which point the actinomycin treated cultures began to deviate from the controls. But this experimental design has the disadvantage of prolonging the phase of discharge of preformed protein as the gradient between cell and medium is less steep than if the medium is replaced at frequent intervals. As a closed circuit operates *in vivo* such a small gradient may approach the physiological situation more closely.

Table II.   Effect of actinomycin D (200 µg/ml) on the concentration of placental proteins in the culture medium after incubation of explants for 24 hours. Figures are the mean and standard deviation of 5 replicate cultures, each 0.5 gm tissue taken from a pool of 10 placentae

	SP_1 ng/ml	PAPP-A IU/ml	hCG IU/ml
Control	1511 ± 81	0.50 ± 0.1	118 ± 14
Actinomycin	2197 ± 804	1.18 ± 0.63	152 ± 8

Table III.   Effect of actinomycin D (200 µg/ml) on the concentration of placental proteins in the culture medium after incubation of explants for 48 hours. Figures are the mean and standard deviation of 5 replicate cultures, each 0.5 gm tissue taken from a pool of 10 placentae

	SP_1 ng/ml	PAPP-A IU/ml	hCG IU/ml
Control	1650 ± 532	0.64 ± 0.22	169 ± 4
Actinomycin	1519 ± 186	0.9 ± 0.29	136 ± 6

CONCLUSIONS

At first glance the data displayed in Figure 7 might suggest that the stage when protein release is dominated by discharge of preformed protein is brief; roughly six hours. It might be pointed out that such findings are based on starting the experiment with a blank medium - that is to say, with a high gradient, much steeper than that which obtains *in vivo*. If one calculates the new release hour by hour starting from a baseline at six hours it is small. It is unlikely that any agent which suppresses biosynthesis only will have a dramatic effect upon protein release in the first 24 or 48 hours, by which time explant cultures are at the end of their physiological lifetime and cotyledon perfusions are long past. Agents which stimulate biosynthesis are likely to be in no better case. It would appear that these short term *in vitro* preparations are better adapted to examining agents which affect the discharge of preformed protein.

The choice between perfusion, explants, cell culture or membrane superfusion depends on the purpose of the experiment. So does whether the medium should be replaced frequently or whether the released products should be allowed to accumulate. No one model or single mode of operation can always produce the best results. In general frequent serial observations give more information than interrupted static observations. Single measurements at relatively long intervals tell nothing about what went on during that interval. The release during a short part of that interval may determine the value for the whole interval obscuring important, but smaller, changes at other times. Discharge of formed protein and fresh biosynthesis take place simultaneously, but the balance changes in favour of the latter as the experiment proceeds. To examine a factor presumed to affect transport or membrane penetration it would be better to concentrate on the early stages of the model's operation. Changes in biosynthesis are more evident later, particularly when the model is operating at near equilibrium conditions because of accumulation of proteins in the medium.

Each technique has its own advantages and disadvantages. Dual perfusion works with an intact placenta and is presumably closer to the *in vivo* state than the culture of explants or dispersed cells. Dual perfusion covers only a short time, although techniques for lengthening this period are now being developed.[16] At present it is more suitable for looking at events concerned with the release of formed protein than at new biosynthesis. Studies on fetal membranes, like dual perfusion, can be done with either open or closed circuit and are simpler to do. Explant culture would appear at first glance to be limited to the equivalent of closed circuit techniques, although frequent sampling will go some way toward a continuous record while still allowing accumulation of protein. Perifusion of separated cells[17] would appear to create the possibility of operating cultures in either a static or a dynamic fashion.

Acknowledgements

Our role in the experimental work on which this review is based is limited to the assay of placental proteins. The dual perfusion experiments were carried out by Dr. Page and his team in Aberdeen. The fetal membrane studies were done by Dr. Mulder and Dr. de Bakker-Teunissen in Amsterdam and the explant cultures by the team working with Dr. Olga Genbacev in Belgrade.

REFERENCES

1. Gordon, Y.B. and Chard, T. (1979) The specific proteins of the human placenta: some new hypotheses. In: "Placental Proteins". Editors: A.

Klopper and T. Chard. Springer Verlag, Heidelberg, pp 1-21.

2. Chard, T. (1986) Placental synthesis. In: "The Human Placenta". Editor: T. Chard, W. B. Saunders, London, pp 447-468.

3. Maruo, T., Matsuo, H., Oishi, T., Hayashi, M., Nishino, R. and Mochizuki, M. (1987) Induction of differentiated trophoblast function by epidermal growth factor: relation of immunohistologically detected epidermal growth factor receptor levels. *J. Clin. Endocrinol. Metab.* **64**, 744-750.

4. Siler-Khoder, T.M., Khoder, G.S., Valenzuela, G. and Rhode, J. (1986) Gonadotropin-releasing hormone effects on placental hormones during gestation: 1. Alpha-human chorionic gonadotropin, human chorionic gonadotropin and human chorionic somatomammotropin. *Biol. Reprod.* **34**, 245-254.

5. Abramovich, D.R., Dacke, C.G., Elcock, C. and Page, K. (1987) Calcium transport across the isolated dually perfused human placental lobule. *J. Physiol.* **382**, 397-410.

6. Panigel, M. (1986) Anatomy and morphology. In: "The Human Placenta". Editor: T. Chard, W.B. Saunders, London, pp 421-446.

7. Ussing, H.H. and Zerahn, K. (1951) Active transport of sodium as the source of an electric current in the short-circuited isolated frog skin. *Acta Physiol. Scand.* **23**, 110-120.

8. Aherne, W. and Dunnill, M.S. (1966) Morphometry of the placenta. *Br. Med. Bull.* **22**, 5-9.

9. Horne, C.H., Towler, C.M., Pugh-Humphreys, R.G.P, Thomson, A.W. and Bohn, H. (1976) Pregnancy specific β_1-glycoprotein. A product of the syncytiotrophoblast. *Experientia* **32**, 1197-1199.

10. Palade, G. (1975) Intracellular aspects of the process of protein synthesis. *Science* **189**, 347-358.

11. Handwerger, S., Wilson, S., Tyrey, L. and Conn, P. (1987) Biochemical evidence that human placental lactogen and chorionic gonadotrophin are not stored in cytoplasmic granules. *Biol. Reprod.* **37**, 28-33.

12. Johnson, S.A. and Wooding, F.B. (1988) Synthesis and storage of chorionic gonadotrophin and placental lactogen in human syncytiotrophoblast *J. Physiol.* **44**, 50.

13. Douglas, W.W. (1968) Stimulus-secretion coupling: the concept and clues from chromaffin and other cells. *Br. J. Pharmacol.* **34**, 451- 474.

14. Bersinger, N.A., Schneider, H. and Keller, P.J. (1986) Synthesis of placental proteins by the human placenta perfused *in vitro*. *Gynecol. Obstet. Invest.* **22**, 47-51.

15. Bischof, P., DuBerg, S., Sizonenko, M., Schineller, A., Beguin, F., Hermann, W. and Sizonenko, P. (1984) *In vitro* production of pregnancy-associated plasma protein A (PAPP-A) by human decidua and trophoblast. *Am. J. Obstet. Gynecol.* **148** 13-19.

16. Miller, R.K., Weir, P.J., Maulik, D. and di Sant'Agnese, P.A. (1985) Human placenta *in vitro*: characterisation during 12 hours of dual perfusion. *Contrib. Gynecol. Obstet.* **13**, 77-84.

17. Sane, A., Harman, I., Quarfordt, S., Costello, A. and Handwerger, S. (1988) Characterisation of placental lactogen release from perifused human trophoblast cells. *Placenta* **9**, 129-138.

As a technique for studying the placenta, simply pumping fluid through the fetal vasculature is unsatisfactory and has been replaced by dual systems, involving simultaneous perfusion of the fetal side through the umbilical vessels and of the maternal side through the intervillous space. But in the delivered placenta there are no convenient single entry and exit points to the intervillous space as there are to the fetal circulation. We are obliged to resort to the clumsy device of puncturing the basal plate and perfusing the intervillous space of a single cotyledon. This brings a host of difficulties in its train. How representative is a single cotyledon? How well do the fetal and maternal perfusion areas match up? How much seepage of maternal fluid into adjacent cotyledons occurs?

In the discussion the mechanics of the enterprise were closely examined. It became clear this is a technique that takes a good workshop and some skill just to build the apparatus; years of trial and error - with a good deal of the latter - have to be endured before satisfactory runs can be obtained consistently. The tricks of technique were well known to our experienced company, so it did not take long for the discussion to pass from the mechanical to the physiological.

How closely does the model reflect the function of the placenta *in vivo*? It depends, of course, on what function you are examining. Perfusion was designed initially to examine the passage of molecules from mother to fetus and vice versa. For this purpose it works moderately well, but there are deficiencies, about which some doubts were expressed. Perfusion fluid is not blood, but attempts to approach the character of blood by adding Dextran, protein, serum or even whole blood have not produced notably successful results. The intact organism holds a great many physiological variables in dynamic balance. The investigator isolates a few, such as flow rate, filtration pressure, oxygenation and pH, and tries to keep them constant. It was agreed that in terms of energy metabolism the dual perfusion preparation is a poor model, however rigorously the known variables are controlled. Fortunately many of the functions we wish to study - such as the synthesis of protein hormones - are robust, and most discussants considered that the release of proteins such as hCG during perfusion was akin to the process *in vivo*.

Much of the criticism levelled at the perfusion model turned about the point of tissue viability. In Rochester a set of working criteria for viability has been evolved, and these criteria were not challenged. Indeed, their fulfilment is a sine qua non before any valid conclusions can be drawn from perfusion experiments. This exposes another disadvantage of the dual perfusion technique. The Rochester group reported keeping a placental cotyledon viable - using their criteria - for up to 12 hours, but the preparation is operated under unphysiological anoxic conditions. Other investigators were agreed that with the usual technique of bubbling 95%

oxygen and 5% carbon dioxide through the perfusion fluid the maximum physiological life of the preparation was three hours; too short a period for many experiments.

A major disadvantage of dual perfusion vis-a-vis other *in vitro* techniques such as superfusion or tissue culture is that true simultaneous controls are not possible. Alternate tests and control periods, reported by participants from Aberdeen, are a poor substitute. Dual perfusion has the advantage of dealing with an intact organ, but the reliability of data on the changes within the tissue itself is open to question. Obviously it is not possible to take tissue samples before perfusion from the cotyledon that is to be perfused. Doubts were expressed about the comparability of samples that perforce must be taken from different areas of the placenta and about the state of the trophoblast after three hours of perfusion.

Two modes of perfusion are possible. One is closed circuit where the perfusion fluid is recycled, allowing the products released by the placenta to accumulate. The other is an open circuit where the perfusing fluid is drained away after one passage through the cotyledon. At first it might appear that the information obtained by either method was much the same. However as discussion proceeded it became clear there were fundamental differences, depending on whether the concentration of placental products in the perfusion fluid had any effect on the placental function being studied. At first glance the closed circuit mimics the physiological situation more closely, but an open circuit appears to present the possibility of measuring the production rate directly. This would be the situation if a steady state was reached where the product was released as fast as it is made. Unfortunately the release of all the proteins - as measured by colleagues from Aberdeen - continued to fall throughout the experiment, and there was no evidence of a steady baseline from which stimulation or suppression of release could be detected easily.

This led to some discussion on the nature of the process studied when the release of protein hormones into the perfusion fluid was measured. Is this simply the discharge of preformed material from the cytoplasm of the trophoblast cell or is the release rate determined by the biosynthesis of fresh protein? Participants from Switzerland and Scotland all produced firm evidence of biosynthesis during the perfusion procedure, but could not say whether it was biosynthesis or discharge mechanisms which determined the release rate.

In the design of perfusion experiments the contents of the perfusion fluid is critical. If the presence or concentration of any placental product in the perfusion fluid affects the release of the substance being measured, closed circuit must be the appropriate mode. These considerations led to the consensus that to get a dynamic picture of the changes in release rate the optimal design in most cases would be a closed circuit sampled frequently.

Definition of terms lies at the heart of communication. It was agreed that "biosynthesis" should be used to designate the assembly of components into an end product - for example, amino acids into polypeptide: "discharge" for the passage of formed product through the plasmalemma, and "secretion" the whole process from biosynthesis, transport within the cell and discharge. "Release" would be applied to what could be observed in the perfusion fluid by measuring the concentration of particular substances. Release is the proper uncommitted term to apply to what is observed in most perfusion experiments where you do not know whether you are dealing with discharge or biosynthesis or both.

PLACENTAL CULTURE

EDITORIAL INTRODUCTION

Turning now from the perfusion of the full term intact placenta, investigation at the cellular level by culture of the trophoblast at any stage of gestation is the next consideration. Both tissue and spheroid cultures can serve as models for the investigation of specific aspects of cell metabolism.

In cell culture, the main advantage is homogeneity of the sample. It is therefore possible to measure release in terms of the number of cells involved. Tissue explants, on the other hand, have the advantage that the anatomical and physiological integrity of the tissue, including cell interaction, is maintained.

So far as the new technique of spheroidal culture is concerned it is appealing because it appears to combine the advantages of both these techniques.

In culture, the medium is the message. The question then arises – how far should media be standardised? Here the problem of comparing the results of different groups of workers rears its head. The problem of standardisation of fetal calf serum has been raised over and over again but not yet solved. One possible solution is the use of well-defined media – but then of course we must know what they should contain in each experimental situation.

Cell cultures can be static – closed – or dynamic – open – which increases the possibilities of getting results likely to help us understand *in vivo* processes, an essential feature of such investigations. The use of culture is primarily to study synthesis and regulation; neither is possible *in vivo*.

From the practical point of view there are some attractive features about culture. Cells can be frozen and live to grow another day, and a competent technician can carry out these procedures with consistently reproducible results.

Finally, what are the clinical situations where culture studies can be of value? Cell-to-cell interaction and cell-to-matrix interaction can tell us a great deal about normal implantation and about invasion by malignant trophoblast.

THE TROPHOBLAST IN SPHEROID CULTURE

Tacey E. White, Risa A. Saltzman, P. Anthony di Sant'Agnese, Robert Sutherland and Richard K. Miller

University of Rochester, Rochester, New York, USA

The *in vitro* culture of trophoblast cells has provided the opportunity to study a wide array of biochemical and physiological functions of the placenta. The development of choriocarcinoma cell lines, in particular JAr, has permitted direct comparison of function with normal cell lines in both terms of morphology and endocrinology.[1] Studies on the control and expression of hormones - for example, human chorionic gonadotrophin, 17 β-oestradiol, and progesterone - have advanced the field of reproductive endocrinology.[2-12]

Unfortunately, with any technique there are limitations. Usually, with monolayer cultures after confluence of the cells there is alteration of normal function. Thus, endocrine function can usually be assessed for periods of a week or less. Furthermore, repeated trypsinisation has also been shown to impair the production of human chorionic gonadotrophin by JAr cells in monolayer culture.[13] Examining morphological interactions between monolayer cultures is also difficult.

To extend the characterisation of trophoblast in culture for longer periods of study - sometimes in excess of three weeks - and in a three dimensional form, a trophoblast multicellular spheroid culture was developed. Other types of tumour cells have already been grown in spheroid culture to examine tumour formation, growth, and response to chemotherapeutic regimens.[14,15] Since spheroids are grown in suspension, growth is not limited by the size of the vessel. Many of these spheroids exceed one mm in diameter. In addition to the same criteria used for monolayer culture, which include morphology, cell proliferation, and endocrine function, attachment or outgrowth of cells can be examined without the use of trypsin.

The current investigation was undertaken to determine if JAr cells could be cultured in a three dimensional state. Such an arrangement would provide the opportunity to examine differentiation, endocrine function, attachment, and the interaction of trophoblast with other types of tissues such as endometrium, in a co-culture system.

The culture methods summarised here are reported in detail elsewhere,[16] and are adapted from spheroid tumour models.[14] JAr choriocarcinoma cells were grown in monolayer culture under the following conditions: RPMI-1640 medium (Gibco), supplemented with 10% fetal calf serum, 1% glutamine, 1%

penicillin-streptomycin, and 1% sodium bicarbonate; humidified 5% CO_2/95% air at 37° C. From these monolayer cultures the trophoblast cells were isolated for spheroid culture.

To develop spheroid cultures, the monolayers of JAr cells were dispersed with trypsin (0.005%) in 0.02% EDTA. The trophoblast cells (5.5 x 10^5 cells in 10 ml of medium) were seeded on to 2% agar-coated LabTek dishes. The cells were incubated for five days in 5% CO_2/95% air at 37° C. During this period the cells divided and formed spheroids. These day-5 spheroids were sized and then seeded into Bellco flasks (500 ml) containing magnetic stir bars and 300 ml of culture medium. Each flask was gassed with 3% CO_2/97% air, sealed, and placed on a magnetic plate in a room at 37° C, and stirred at 110 rpm. Between days nine and 11 the flasks were transferred to stir plates at 190 rpm. Such a change is necessary because of the size and weight of the spheroids. The medium was changed every 48 hours.

Radioimmunoassays of human chorionic gonadotrophin, 17 β-oestradiol, and progesterone were performed on the medium to determine the rate of hormone release per spheroid per 48 hours (hCG - Tandem R; E_2 - Leeco; P_4 - Diagnostic Products).

The mean size of each spheroid group was determined by measuring two perpendicular diameters on each of 30 spheroids. A geometric mean diameter (GMD) and standard deviation was then calculated for each group. Spheroid volume was calculated using the equation:

$$V = (4/3) (GMD/2)^3$$

Morphological assessments of the spheroids were performed with light and electron microscopy (transmission and scanning). For light microscopy, JAr spheroids were fixed in 10% phosphate-buffered formalin (pH 7.3), embedded in paraffin, and stained with haematoxylin and eosin. Spheroids for transmission and scanning electron microscopy were fixed as previously described.[16,17]

To assess attachment and outgrowth on to a surface by the spheroids, the spheroids were placed into a 60 mm plastic culture dish in 5 ml of supplemented medium for either five to six days or 12 to 15 days in 5% CO_2/95% air at 37° C. The contents were stained with methylene blue, and spheroid attachment and growth of cells assessed using an inverted light microscope. The standard for outgrowth was the day-5 spheroid, which attached and grew out on to culture dishes to a distance at least equal to its radius.

DISCUSSION OF THE RESULTS

Multicellular spheroids were consistently formed from JAr choriocarcinoma cells, and these spheroids were maintained in culture for at least three weeks. The shape and size of the spheroids varied with length of incubation. Initially, young spheroids ranged from spherical to very irregular in shape. Individual cells could be distinguished at the periphery of the spheroid. After several days of culture, the spheroids became more defined and spherical in shape with the outer cells becoming flattened. Comparisons of JAr spheroids with monolayer cultures showed a similar cellular morphology (Figs. 1 and 2). The spheroid cells were anaplastic with a relatively high nuclear to cytoplasmic ratio. Mitotic figures were present, with some appearing pleomorphic. By day 7 (Fig. 2a-b), scattered cells showed evidence of aptotic necrosis. Day-15 spheroids were very similar in appearance to day-7 spheroids (Fig. 2c-d). The shape

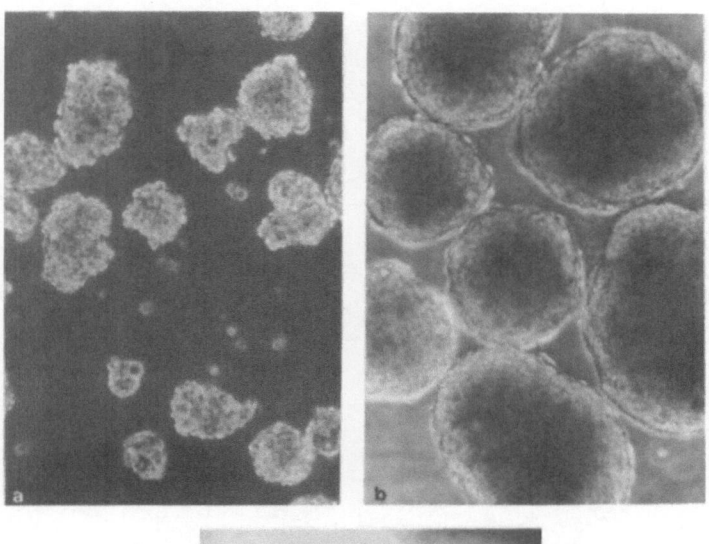

Figure 1.   JAr spheroids in plastic culture dishes during medium
changes on a) day 7 (205.3 ± 17.0 μ), b) day 11 (497.2
± 64.2 μ) and c) day 17 of culture (948.2 ± 73.3 μ).

was well defined, and the spheroid was composed of tightly packed
arrangements of cells. By day 15, aptotic necrotic cells appeared with
small areas of focal necrosis (or empty spaces), which may have been where
degenerated cells once were. However, there was no central necrotic core
present on day 15 as has often been noted for other tumour-cell spheroids
(Fig. 2a-d)[14,15,18,19] Such lack of a necrotic core for the trophoblast
cells is attributed to the known anaerobic energy capabilities of the
trophoblast.[20-22] By 21 days the spheroids began to lose their spherical
shape and became quite flattened. Such flattening was attributed to the
appearance and increase in size of a central necrotic core.

Classic spheroid morphology includes a viable, mitotically active outer
layer of cells, a less densely stained intermediate zone, and a central
core of necrosis.[13] In other spheroid systems, this central necrotic core
begins developing when the diameter of the spheroid is less than 400μ.[14,]

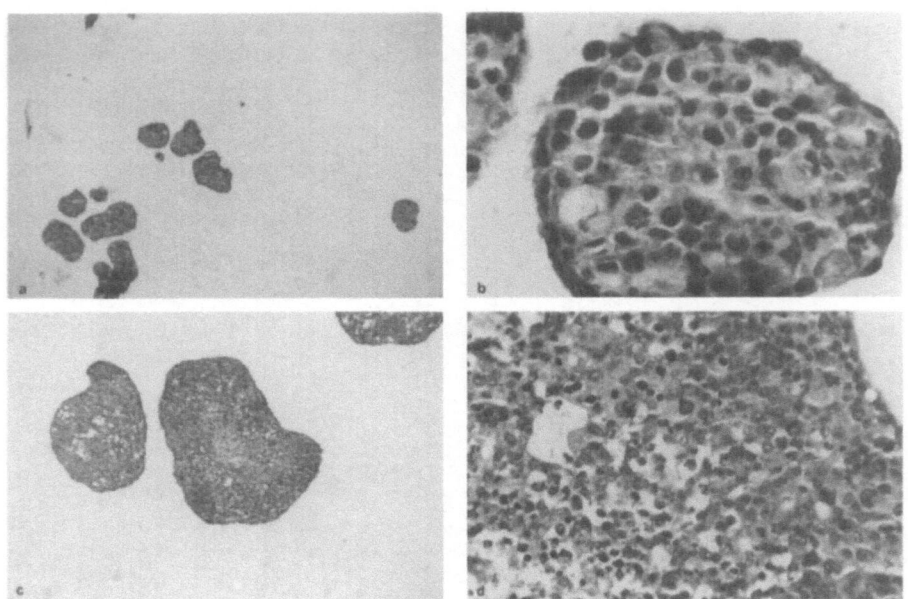

Figure 2.   Morphology of day-7 and day-15 JAr spheroids

a-b   Day-7 spheroids. Generally, cells are anaplastic with
            moderate to high nuclear cytoplasmic ratios. Cell
            nuclei are round, hyperchromatic and usually contain a
            single large amphophilic nucleolus. Scattered cells
            undergo aptotic necrosis; no central necrotic core is
            noted. a) 54X, b) 600X.

c-d   Day-15 spheroids: very similar to day 7, except for
            increased size and more aptotic necrotic cells. Note
            especially absence of a central necrotic core, which is
            not generally seen until diameter exceeds 1 mm (not
            shown). c) 54X, d) 600X.

[18,19,23] Interestingly, no JAr spheroids of less than 900µ diameter had a
central necrotic core. The JAr spheroids were characterised by a thick,
viable outer layer of cells and an intermediate zone with mitotic figures
throughout. It should be noted that in the absence of a central necrotic
core the trophoblast spheroids continued to show small focal areas of
absent cells or necrosis surrounded by areas of viable cells within the
intermediate zone. This adaptation to anaerobic conditions may reflect the
relatively hypoxic conditions in utero.

    On day 5, the trophoblast spheroids have a GMD of 125 ± 8.8µ with a
calculated volume of 0.001 mm³. When these day-5 spheroids are seeded into
the flasks both the GMD and the volume increase logarithmically with
respect to days in culture (Fig. 3). By 21 days, spheroid size was at a
plateau between 1100 and 1300µ.

    The ultrastructure of the JAr spheroid consisted of a cytoplasm
characterised by polyribosome rosettes and short strands of rough and
smooth endoplasmic reticulum (Fig. 4). Scattered lipid droplets and rounded
patches of apparently nonstaining glycogen were present in some of the
cells. Small to moderate numbers of mitochondria were also present, as well
as scattered cytoplasmic arrays of annulate lamellae (White et al,

86

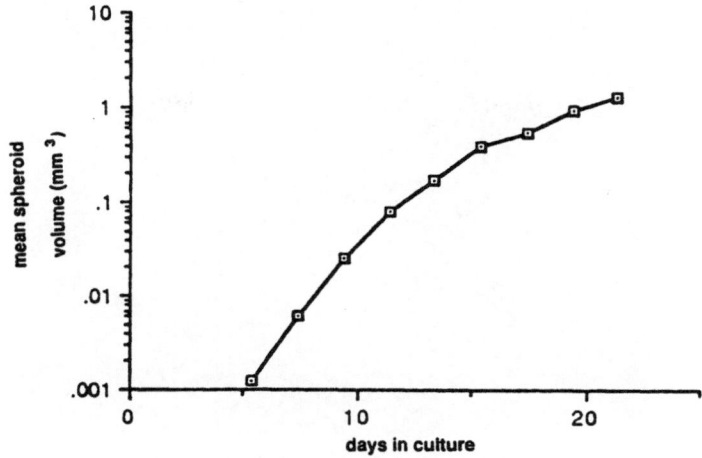

Figure 3.   Spheroid   growth: volume   increased in linear fashion
             with days in culture.

unpublished data).   The   intercellular spaces were wide, with prominent
microvilli projecting into them.   Microvilli were also present on the outer
surface of the spheroids.   Primitive cell to cell junctions, possibly gap
junctions,   were seen.   Up to day 15, the spheroids continued to maintain a
similar ultrastructural appearance,   but the cells appeared to have fewer
microvilli.   The Golgi complex appeared prominent in some of the cells,
which also contained larger, more atypical, mitochondria. The outer cells
varied widely in size with microvilli being numerous on the surface of the
spheroid (Fig. 4).

    The spheroids produced increasing (linear with respect to volume of the
spheroid) amounts of human chorionic gonadotrophin, 17 β-oestradiol, and
progesterone as expressed per spheroid per 48 hours (Fig.   5).   When the
spheroids exceed 1 mm³ in volume, human chorionic gonadotrophin release was
> 100 mIU/spheroid/48 hours;   oestradiol was > 70 pg/spheroid/48 hours;
progesterone was 29 ng/spheroid/48 hours.   The increase in hormone release
was linearly related to spheroid volume. Hormone secretion correlated best
with spheroid size rather than simply time in culture.   Certainly the
hormone secretion by the JAr spheroid is similar to monolayer cultures,
even though direct comparisons are difficult to make.   Preliminary results
indicate that the histochemical localisation of human chorionic gonadotrophin within the spheroid is positive in approximately 25% of the cells, but
not localised to any specific region of the spheroid.   These observations
are consistent with the observation that cells with the cytotrophoblastic
phenotype produce human chorionic gonadotrophin to a much smaller extent
than syncytiotrophoblast cells.[24-26] Since 1-5% of cells in the spheroids
stained darkly with antibodies against human chorionic gonadotrophin it
appears that these cells exist in different states of functional maturity
within the spheroid or there may be variations in the cellular phenotypes
within the JAr cell line itself.

    The ability of the JAr cells to grow out from spheroids on to plastic
dishes was assessed as another measure of spheroid cell function.   Day-5
spheroids attached to the plastic dishes began to demonstrate cellular
outgrowth within 24 hours. After five to six days, these spheroids
exhibited an outgrowth which extended to a distance equal to their own
radius (Fig. 6a).   The outgrowth consisted of single or multiple layers of
JAr cells having a cytotrophoblastic phenotype.   After 12 to 15 days in

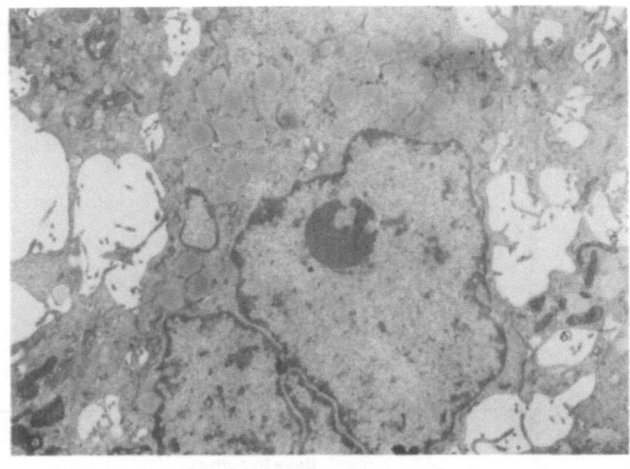

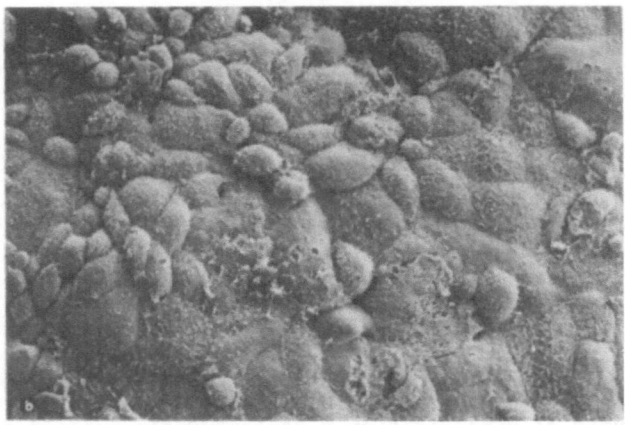

Figure 4.   a) Electromicrograph of a day-5 JAr spheroid. Note wide
intercellular spaces with prominent microvilli, also
present along outer surface of scattered lipid droplets
in some cells; primitive cell-to-cell junctions,
possibly gap junctions (500X).

b) Scanning electronmicrograph from a day 17 JAr
spheroid. Note the tightly-packed surface cells, size
variations, and numerous microvilli (1800X).

culture, the spheroids produced a more extensive, multilayered outgrowth,
containing cells which in general retained a cytotrophoblastic phenotype.
There were an occasional bi- and multinucleated cell or cells with
cytoplasmic projections along the edge of the outgrowth (Fig. 6b-c). JAr
spheroids of up to 700μ in diameter (day 15) attached and grew out on to
culture dishes to an extent comparable with day-5 spheroids. By contrast,
spheroids with a diameter greater than 800μ attached to culture plates, but
did not produce cell extension over the entire circumference. Usually,
outgrowth was limited to one section or area only. In the day-21 spheroid
(approximately 1200μ) both attachment and outgrowth was impaired. After
five to six days in outgrowth culture their activity came to a halt.
However, by days 12 to 15 the spheroids appeared to regain their ability to
attach and grow out. The monolayers of outgrowth from these large spheroids
showed more cellular projections and tendency to be multinuclear than the
comparable outgrowth from day-5 spheroids.

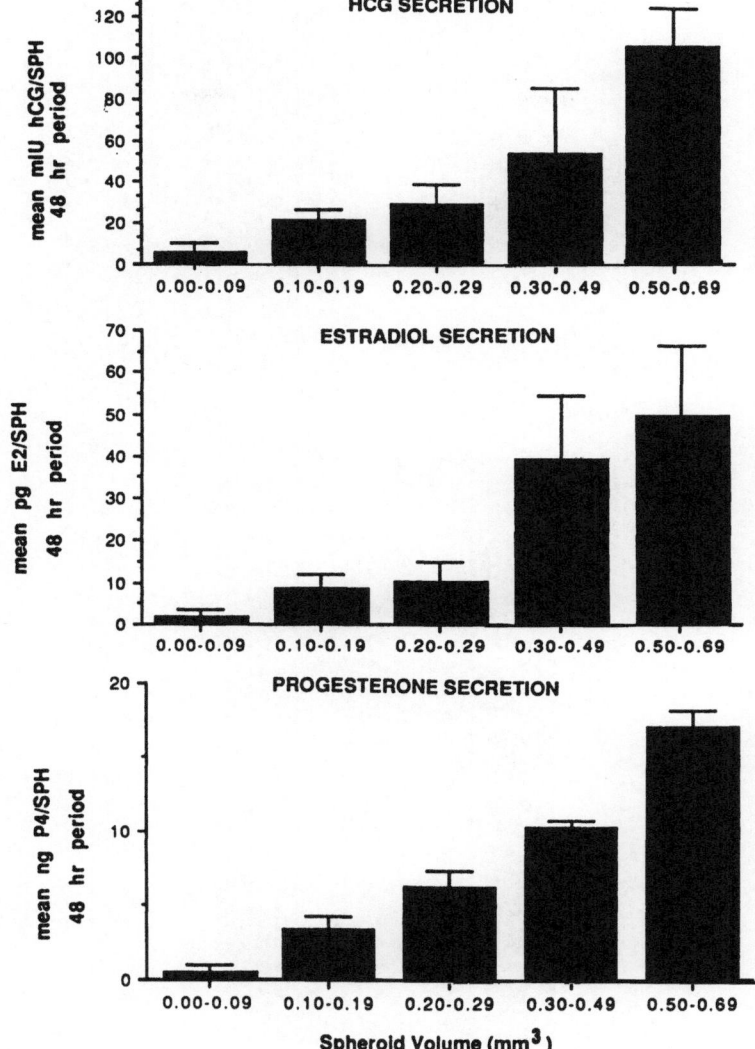

Figure 5. Hormone secretion. Secretion into medium on a per
spheroid basis during a 48-hr period increased with
volume of spheroid. a) Human chorionic gonadotrophin
(mIU hCG/spheroid/48 hours), b) 17 β-oestradiol (pg E_2/
spheroid/48 hours) and c) progesterone (ng P_4/spheroid/
48 hours).

These changes of ability to grow out in the larger JAr spheroids are
inconsistent with other spheroid systems, where outgrowth capability is
present even when the diameter exceeds 1200μ.[15] Since JAr spheroids of 800μ
did not uniformly have a distinct necrotic core, the impaired ability to
grow out cannot be attributed to lack of cellular viability. The changes in
outgrowth may simply represent a change in cell function along the
periphery of the trophoblast spheroid. Such a possibility is supported by
the observation that very large spheroids, which initially did not grow
out, eventually regained this ability. Furthermore, in the outgrowth of
these larger spheroids, there were more areas of bi- and multinucleated
cells with granular cytoplasm, projections, and evidence of sprouting. All

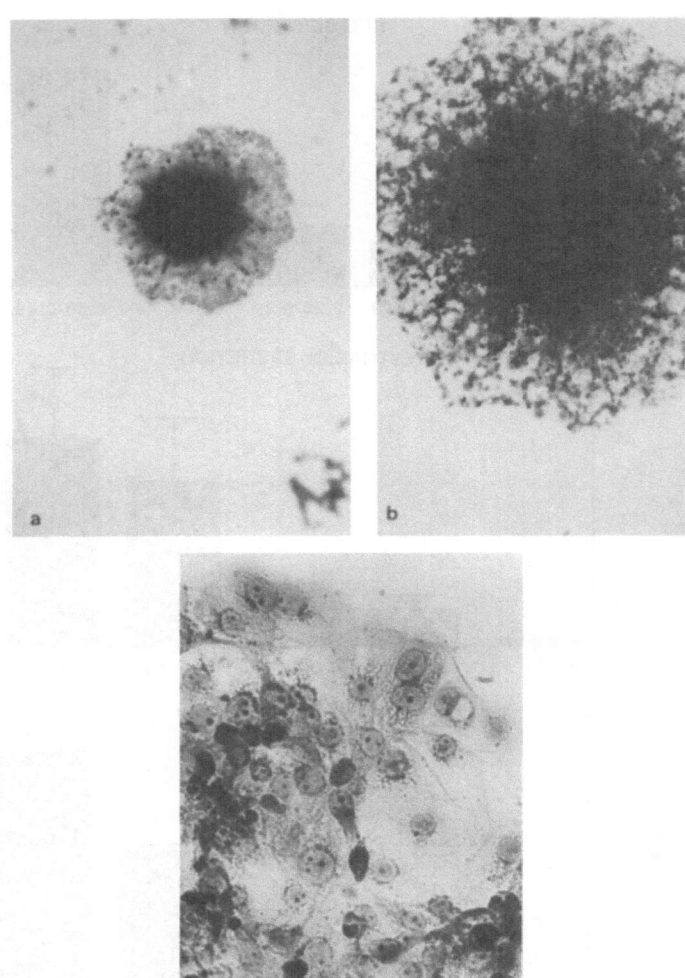

Figure 6.   Outgrowth of 5 day JAr spheroids onto culture dishes.
a) Outgrowth after 5-6 days. b) Outgrowth after 12-15
days. c) Outgrowth after 12-15 days. Note morphological
characteristics and limited multinuclearity (375X).

of these characteristics are consistent with the differentiation of normal
trophoblast.[20,26]

Such manipulations of the trophoblast, which do not require enzymatic
dispersal, give additional opportunities to study normal function. The
outgrowth studies may reflect some of the phenomena of invasion and
implantation.   Three-dimensional cellular interactions such as differentiation and implantation can be adapted from this spheroid system because
there is an extended culture period of at least 21 days, there are large
and free cellular masses for easy manipulation, the shape better reflects
the state of the trophoblast mass *in vivo* than does monolayer culture, and
there are large numbers of cells generated from each experiment.

Acknowledgements

Dr. Ronald Pattillo of the Medical College of Wisconsin kindly provided the JAr cells for this study. Dr. David Penney of the University of Rochester performed the transmission electron microscopy, and Karen Demesy-Jensen provided technical assistance with same. This research was supported in part by National Institutes of Health grants ES02774, ES01247, CA11198, and CA11051.

REFERENCES

1. Pattillo, R.A., Ruckert, A., Hussa, R.O., Bernstein, R. and Delfs, E. (1971) The JAr cell line: continuous human multihormone production and controls. *In Vitro* **6**, 398–399.
2. Pattillo, R.A. and Gey, G.O. (1968) The establishment of a cell line of human hormone-synthesising trophoblastic cells *in vitro*. *Cancer Res.* **28**, 1231–1236.
3. Bridson, W.E., Ross, G.T. and Kohler, P.O. (1971) Immunologic and biologic activity of chorionic gonadotrophin synthesised by cloned choriocarcinoma cells in culture. *J. Clin. Endocrinol. Metab.* **33**, 145–149.
4. Pattillo, R.A., Hussa, R.O., Huang, W.Y., Delfs, E. and Mattingly, R.F. (1972) Estrogen production of trophoblastic tumours in tissue culture. *J. Clin. Endocrinol. Metab.* **34**, 59–61.
5. Bellino, F.L., Hussa, R.O. and Osawa, Y. (1978) Estrogen synthetase in choriocarcinoma cell culture. Stimulation by dibutyryl cyclic adenosine monophosphate and theophyline. *Steroids* **32**, 37–44.
6. Hussa, R.O., Story, M.T., Pattillo, R.A. and Kemp, R.A. (1977) Effect of cyclic 3':5'-AMP derivatives, prostaglandins and related agents on human chorionic gonadotrophin secretion in human malignant trophoblast in culture. *In Vitro* **13**, 443–449.
7. Benveniste, R., Speeg, K.V. jun, Carpenter, G., Cohen, S., Lindner, J. and Rabinowitz, D. (1978) Epidermal growth factor stimulates secretion of human chorionic gonadotropin by cultured human choriocarcinoma cells. *J. Clin. Endocrinol. Metab.* **46**, 169–172.
8. Story, M.T., Hussa, R.O. and Pattillo, R.A. (1974) Independent dibutyryl cyclic adenosine monophosphate stimulation of human chorionic gonadotropin and estrogen secretion by malignant trophoblast cells *in vitro*. *J. Clin. Endocrinol. Metab.* **39**, 877–881.
9. Bahn, R.S., Worsham, A., Speeg, K.V. jun, Ascoli, M. and Rabin, D. (1981) Characterisation of steroid production in cultured human choriocarcinoma cells. *J. Clin. Endocrinol. Metab.* **52** (3), 447–450.
10. Browne, P. and Bagshawe, K.D. (1982) Enhancement of human chorionic gonadotrophin production by antimetabolites. *Br. J. Cancer.* **46**, 22–29.
11. Ilekis, J. and Benveniste, R. (1985) Effects of epidermal growth factor, phorbol myristate acetate, and arachidonic acid on choriogonadotropin secretion by cultured human choriocarcinoma cells. *Endocrinology* **116**, 2400–2409.
12. Bellino, F.L. and Hussa, R.O. (1985) Estrogen synthetase stimulation by hemin in human choriocarcinoma cell culture. *Biochem. Biophys. Res. Commun.* **127**, 232–238.
13. Pattillo, R.A., Hussa, R.O., Ruckert, A.C.F., Kurtz, J.W., Cade, J.M. and Rinke, M.L. (1979) Human chorionic gonadotrophin in BeWo trophoblastic cells after 12 years in continuous culture: Retention of intact human chorionic gonadotrophin secretion in mechanically versus enzyme-dispersed cells. *Endocrinology* **105**, 967–974.
14. Sutherland, R.M., McCredie, J.A., and Inch, W.R. (1971) Growth of multicell spheroids in tissue culture as a model of nodular carcinomas. *J. Natl. Cancer. Inst.* **46**, 113–117.

15. Sutherland, R.M. (1988) Cell and environment interactions in tumour microregions: The multicell spheroid model. *Science* **240**, 177-184.
16. White, T.E., Saltzman, R.A, di Sant'Agnese, P.A., Keng, P., Sutherland, R. and Miller, R.K. (1988) Human choriocarcinoma (JAr) cells grown as multicellular spheroids. *Placenta* In press.
17. di Sant'Agnese, P.A., Demesy-Jensen, K., Miller, R.K., Wier, P.J., and Maulik, D. (1987) Long term human placental lobule perfusion – an ultrastructural study. *Trophoblast Res.* **2**, 549-560.
18. Sutherland, R.M. and Durand, R.E. (1973) Hypoxic cells in an *in vitro* tumour model. *Int. J. Radiat. Biol.* **23**, 235-246.
19. Soranzo, C., Torre-Della, G. and Ingrosso, A. (1986) Formation, growth and morphology of multicellular tumor spheroids from human colon carcinoma cell line (LoVo). *Tumorigen* **72**, 459-467.
20. Aladjem, S. and Lueck, J. (1981) Morphologic characteristics of the normal term human trophoblast maintained in prolonged *in vitro* cultures. *Br. J. Obstet. Gynaecol.* **88**, 287-293.
21. Aladjem, S., Lueck, J. and Tsai, A. (1980) A method for the prolonged *in vitro* culture of normal human trophoblast. *Proc. Fed. Am. Soc. Exp. Biol.* **39**, 506.
22. Morgan, D.M.L., Toothill, V.J. and Landon, M.J. (1985) Long-term culture of human trophoblast cells. *Br. J. Obstet. Gynaecol.* **92**, 84-92.
23. Mulcahy, R.T., Rosenkrans, W.A. jun, Penney, D.P. and Cooper, R.A. (1985) The growth and multicellular spheroids *in vitro*. *In Vitro* **21**, 513-519.
24. Speeg, K.V. jun, Azizkhan, J.C. and Stromberg, K. (1976) The stimulation by methotrexate of human chorionic gonadotrophin and placental alkaline phosphatase in cultured choriocarcinoma cells. *Cancer Res.* **36**, 4570-4576.
25. Friedman, S.J. and Skehan, P. (1979) Morphological differentiation of human choriocarcinoma cells induced by methotrexate. *Cancer Res.* **36**, 1960-1967.
26. Kliman, H.J., Feinman, M.A. and Strauss, J.F. (1987) Differentiation of human cytotrophoblast into syncytiotrophoblast in culture. *Trophoblast Res.* **2**, 407-421.

TISSUE EXPLANT TECHNIQUE IN THE STUDY OF HUMAN CHORIONIC GONADOTROPHIN
(hCG) PRODUCTION *IN VITRO*

Bojana Čemerikić and Olga Genbačev

Institute of Endocrinology, Immunology and Nutrition
INEP, Zemun, Yugoslavia

Human chorionic gonadotrophin (hCG) is a glycoprotein hormone normally secreted by trophoblastic cells of the placenta during pregnancy, which signals the differentiation of the trophoblast from the remainder of the blastocyst.

The mechanisms involved in the control of placental hormone production are not yet understood. The human placenta has been considered autonomous in its synthesis and secretion of protein and steroid hormones. The possibility that there are some control factors involved in the regulation of hCG production has been investigated by many workers. A logical candidate for the possible feed-back regulatory agent is progesterone, but it has been shown[1] that progesterone has no effect on hCG secretion by first trimester tissue explants. However, it does inhibit hCG production by first trimester trophoblast cell culture,[2] and a hypothesis has been put forward that progesterone may be a factor involved in the inhibitory regulation of hCG production.[2] At higher concentrations, progesterone suppresses hCG secretion by term placenta explant cultures,[3,4] suggesting that it may be responsible for declining hCG production as gestation advances to term.

The clinical observation that bromocriptine treatment of pregnant women with hyperprolactinaemia results in the decrease of prolactin (PRL) levels with parallel increases in the concentration of serum hCG stimulated studies of possible PRL effect on hCG production *in vitro*. Prolactin inhibits hCG production in term placental explants.[5] The doses of PRL used in these experiments were comparable to the concentrations of PRL present in mother and fetus. In view of the close anatomical relationship of the trophoblast and decidua which synthesises PRL de novo, the possibility of a paracrine regulation of hCG in trophoblast near term was suggested.

During the past ten years a number of peptides once believed to occur only in the hypothalamus have been extracted from placental tissue. Corticotrophin-releasing factor (CRF), thyrotrophin-releasing factor (TRF), luteinising hormone-releasing factor (LH-RF), endorphine-like peptides, and dynorphine have all been reported to be present in the placenta.[6-10] In addition, the presence of receptors specific for LH-RF[11] and opiate binding sites[12-15] has been demonstrated in the syncytiotrophoblast brush border membrane of the human placenta. These facts prompted the study of the possible role of LH-RF and opiate peptides in the autocrine regulation of

93

hCG production. So far it has been shown that LH–RF causes specific stimulation of hCG release *in vitro* in a dose-dependent mode,[16] the maximum occurring in 16–17 weeks old placentae.[17]

The possible role of endogenous opioids in the regulation of hCG has been investigated,[18] and dynorphine shown to stimulate potassium-induced release of hCG in term placental slices perifused *in vitro*. We have reported direct morphine stimulation of hCG release by trophoblast tissue explants from individual early human placentae.[19]

Recently, inhibin, a gonadal glycoprotein hormone, has been identified in the cytotrophoblast layer of human placenta at term and in primary culture of human trophoblasts.[20] It is suggested that inhibin may have an important role in the paracrine regulation of placental hCG production by local tonic inhibitory action.

All information so far available about hCG production and its regulation comes from *in vitro* experiments using cell or tissue culture techniques. Clinical data – connected mostly with the pattern of hCG secretion – give some support to the *in vitro* data.

TISSUE EXPLANT TECHNIQUE

In an attempt to contribute to the understanding of hCG synthesis and its regulation, we have chosen the first trimester trophoblast tissue explant technique as a model for several reasons. Compared to cell culture, this technique offers the following advantages: (a) maintenance of a higher level of biological organisation closer to the *in vivo* situation; (b) differentiated status based on cell-cell and cell-matrix interactions is better preserved; and (c) proteolytic enzymes for cell isolation are unnecessary. The major disadvantages of this technique are that it is difficult to produce homogeneous tissue explants, and the central zone of explants tends to degenerate due to inadequate oxygenation and lack of nutrients. Using tissue explants from first trimester trophoblast reduces these disadvantages, because they consist mostly of "tips" of chorionic villi – that is, syncytiotrophoblast, cytotrophoblast and mesenchymal core. Using the same technique in the preparation of term placental tissue explants is much more difficult because of the complex organisation of villous structure.

How the tissue explant technique should be used depends on what one intends to study. Its major limitation is time; tissue cannot be maintained under *in vitro* conditions for indefinite periods. To establish a maximum duration of the experiment it is necessary to operate strict criteria for checking tissue viability and standardising the system. A variety of different incubation media are commonly used to culture tissue explants, from simple basal medium (Eagle) to more complex media (Medium 199; Ham's F12). This leads to different survival times of the explants, which in turn makes it difficult to compare results from different sources.

We have used two different protocols to culture trophoblast tissue explants: (A) short-term incubation, up to 24 hours, and (B) tissue culture up to 6 days. Protocol A engendered less risk of tissue damage and the effects of an unphysiological situation. Two sets of experiments were conducted to obtain data on hCG release using this experimental approach.

Protocol A

Trophoblast tissue from individual placentae (8–11 weeks gestation) was preincubated for one hour to wash out contaminants, damaged tissue and blood, and then incubated for six hours in McCoy 5a medium. Aliquots (0.1 ml) were withdrawn at one hour intervals and kept frozen until analysed.

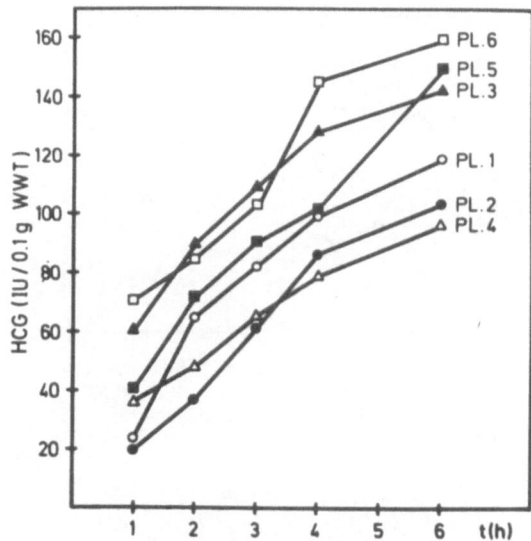

Figure 1. Time course of hCG release by individual first trimester placentae in short-term incubation of trophoblast
tissue explants. The tissue was obtained and incubated
as previously described.[21] hCG determination was performed as described previously.[19] hCG is expressed as
IU/0.1 g wwt. Pl. 1 to Pl. 6. = individual placentae.

The results obtained are summarised in Figure 1. During a six-hour
incubation, the concentration of hCG in the medium increased gradually in
all individual placentae studied. The hCG concentration has been standardised for the weight of tissue in each individual culture. When the results
are expressed in terms of the concentration per 100 mg tissue there is
still considerable variation between different placentae; a phenomenon
which might contribute to the large patient-to-patient differences found in
serum hCG concentrations during normal pregnancy.

To determine whether hCG released into the medium is preformed or newly
synthesised another group of short-term experiments was carried out with
the time extended up to 24 hours, introducing cycloheximide (20 mcg/ml) as
a protein synthesis inhibitor. To measure the effect of cycloheximide, 1 ml
aliquots of incubation media were withdrawn at two-hour intervals. The
amounts of medium taken and replaced by blank medium (5% of total volume)
seemed to be reasonable in terms of not exposing tissue to frequent and
severe changes in the tissue-medium gradient. It can be seen (Fig. 2) that
during a 24-hour incubation, the concentration of hCG in the medium
containing cycloheximide was not significantly different from that in the
control, indicating that most or all of the hCG found in the medium was
preformed. Similar results have been obtained with term placental tissue
explants,[22] suggesting that the hCG biosynthesis during the first 24 hours
of culture is minimal compared to the amount released from preformed
hormone.

From the foregoing we concluded that incubation of placental tissue
explants up to 24 hours can be useful for the study of hCG release and
possible factors and mechanisms involved in its regulation.

Protocol B

To study the rate of hCG biosynthesis *in vitro* it is necessary to
maintain long-term tissue culture of the explants. By measuring hCG

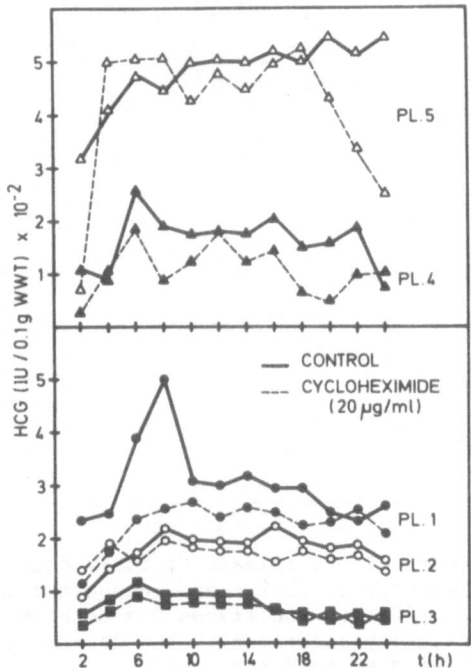

Figure 2. Cycloheximide effect on hCG release by individual first trimester placentae in short-term *in vitro* incubation. Tissue and notation as in Figure 1.

concentration in the medium expressed per unit time and weight of tissue we are estimating hCG production, which takes in biosynthesis, intracellular transport, and secretion. To this end, a culture procedure of trophoblast explants described by Maruo et al[2] was adopted. Trophoblast tissue (50 mcg wet weight) was placed on Whatman filter paper immersed in 2.5 ml of McCoy 5a medium, and incubated up to 144 hours. The length of time of tissue culture was based on two criteria of tissue viability – morphological appearance, and metabolic activity as evidenced by glucose consumption and lactate production.

Figure 3 illustrates the morphological appearance of the tissue incubated for (A) 24, and (B) 144 hours. It can be seen that the trophoblast layer retains its structural integrity after 144 hours of culture.

Glucose consumption and lactate production remained constant throughout the culture period (3.5 ± 0.82 and 0.93 ± 0.05 mg/0.1 g wwt/24 h for glucose and lactate). The pattern of hCG production rate (IU/0.1 g wwt/24 h) is shown on Figure 4. Maximal hCG production rate was observed during the fourth day of culture. From day 4 to day 6, the production rate of hCG remained relatively constant and higher than in the first three days.

The addition of cycloheximide to the culture medium produced a significant inhibitory effect after 48 hours of exposure (Fig. 5, left). The replacement of cycloheximide-containing medium by blank medium after 72 hours (Fig. 5, right) did not restore the ability of the tissue to produce hCG; production remained low relative to the control. The cycloheximide experiments suggest that hCG found in the medium after 48 hours of culture represents newly synthesised hormone. These results are consistent with those obtained by measuring the incorporation of labelled amino acid precursor into the hormone molecule.[2]

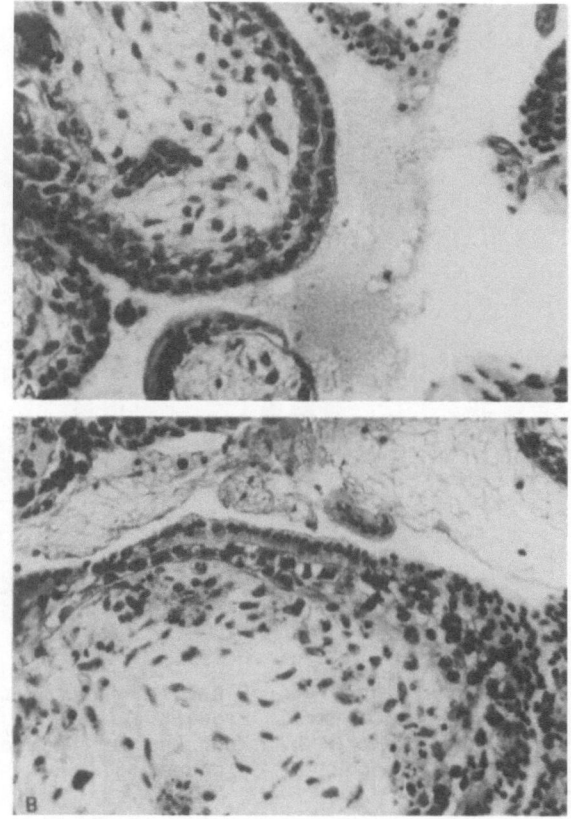

Figure 3.   The morphological appearance of first trimester tropho-
            blast tissue cultured for 24 (A) and 144 hrs (B). Bouin
            fixative; magnification x 640.

In summary, to study the true rate of hCG biosynthesis the tissue
should be maintained *in vitro* for longer than three days. It is important
to check tissue viability when maintaining the culture for maximal
duration. The use of trophoblast tissue from individual placentae greatly
reduces variations in the results, and also makes it possible to use each
placenta as its own control.

MORPHINE EFFECT ON hCG

The validity of protocols A and B in the study of hCG regulation was
tested using morphine and naloxone. Opioids were selected because their
involvement in the regulation of hCG release has already been postulated.[18]

Explants as described above were exposed to morphine and naloxone up to
six hours, and the hCG concentration in the medium was measured. The
results (Table I) show that morphine (100 nM) consistently increases hCG
release in first trimester placentae (n = 16). The effect varied between
individual placentae, ranging from 33% to 181% increases over control
values.

Pretreatment of the tissue with naloxone, in a dose of 100 nM, blocked
the effect of morphine on hCG release (Figs. 6a, 6c). Naloxone itself (Fig.
6b) had no effect on hCG release.

97

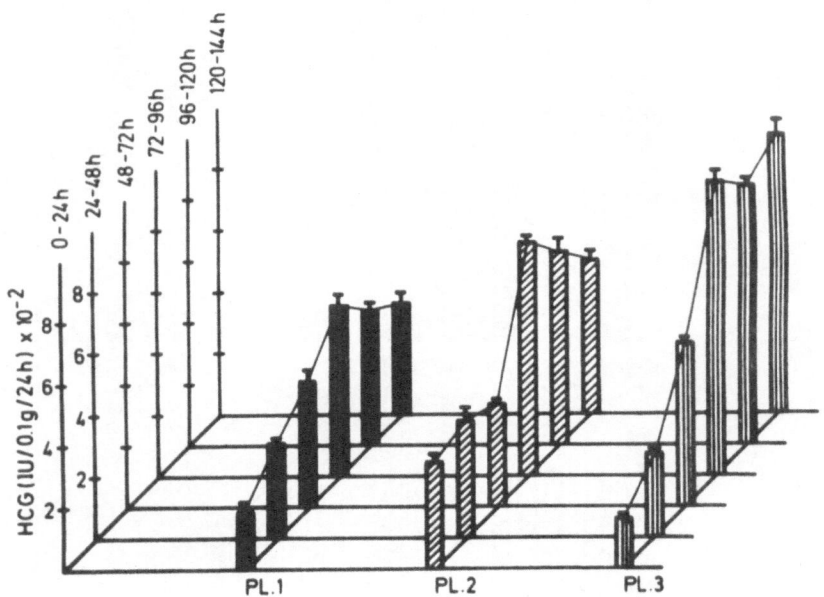

Figure 4. The production rate of hCG in three first trimester placentae in culture. Production rate of hCG expressed as IU/0.1 g wwt/24 h. Each bar is the mean value ± SEM from five independent cultures.

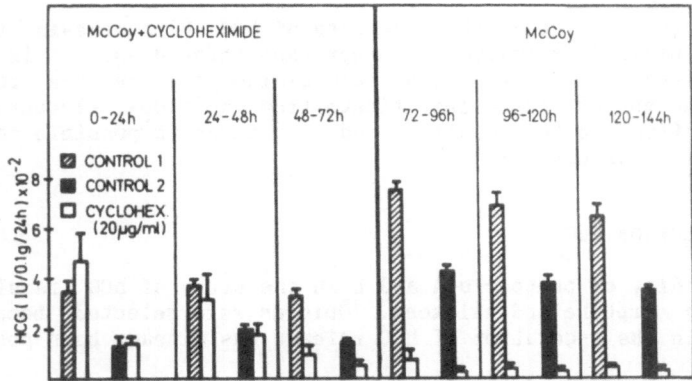

Figure 5. Cycloheximide effect on hCG production rate in two cultures of first trimester trophoblast. Culture as in Figure 4. Controls 1 and 2 are the controls of two individual placentae. Results expressed as IU/0.1 g wwt/24 h. Each bar is the mean value ± SEM from five independent cultures.

Table I. Morphine effect on hCG release in first trimester placentae. Procedure as for Fig. 1. Results expressed as IU/0.1 g wwt. Each value is the mean ± SEM from five independent flasks. Pl. 1 to Pl. 16 = individual placenta

	Control	Morphine (100 nM)	% of Increase
Pl. 1	67.55 ± 1.53	171.5 ± 4.32	153
Pl. 2	58.10 ± 1.58	163.8 ± 1.64	181
Pl. 3	75.33 ± 3.21	130.8 ± 1.64	172
Pl. 4	36.60 ± 6.36	94.5 ± 4.95	158
Pl. 5	130.20 ± 2.65	173.6 ± 3.62	33
Pl. 6	103.14 ± 5.56	145.8 ± 4.40	41
Pl. 7	87.22 ± 1.64	129.7 ± 1.78	48
Pl. 8	111.92 ± 2.36	154.8 ± 5.67	37
Pl. 9	175.90 ± 1.94	240.6 ± 3.77	36
Pl. 10	15.37 ± 3.03	27.4 ± 3.47	78
Pl. 11	34.37 ± 1.87	61.7 ± 0.90	79
Pl. 12	18.48 ± 1.78	35.7 ± 2.19	93
Pl. 13	96.08 ± 2.80	174.1 ± 5.28	81
Pl. 14	53.53 ± 3.92	98.5 ± 2.00	84
Pl. 15	50.00 ± 3.40	95.7 ± 0.70	91
Pl. 16	26.90 ± 0.30	42.1 ± 2.60	55

These short-term experiments show that morphine, in the nanomolar range, increases the release of preformed hCG from first trimester trophoblast tissue explants *in vitro*. This effect was not obtained in explants from term placenta.[19]

To see whether morphine will also affect hCG production rate, long-term tissue culture experiments (Protocol B) were performed. As illustrated in Figure 7, the stimulatory effect of morphine on hCG release was seen again over the first 24 hours. During the second, third and fourth day the production of hCG increased. On days 5 and 6, this effect was no longer detectable.

This stimulation of hCG by morphine (Fig. 8, left) can be reversed by replacing morphine-containing medium with the control medium (Fig. 8, right).

From the foregoing we have seen that morphine consistently stimulates the release of preformed hCG in short-term incubation and in hCG biosynthesis as measured by its production rate in long-term culture of first trimester trophoblast tissue explants. The effect is reversible and can be prevented by pretreatment with naloxone. As the dose of morphine used in

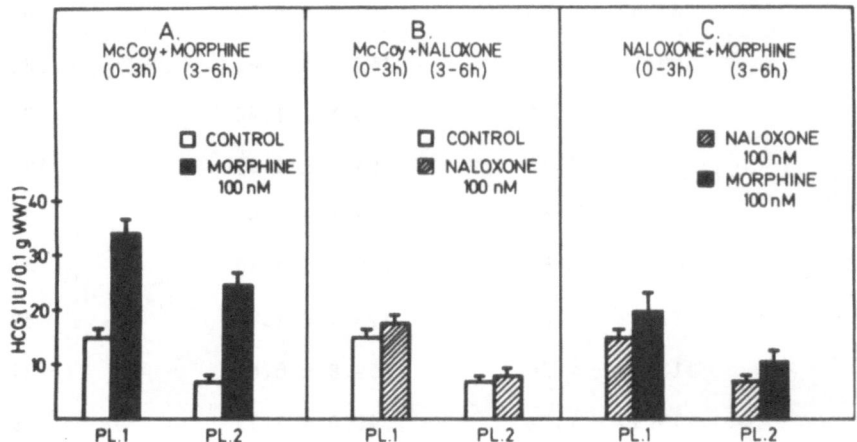

Figure 6.   Effect of morphine and naloxone on hCG release in first trimester placentae. Results expressed as IU/0.1 g wwt. Each bar is the mean ± SEM from five independent incubation flasks.

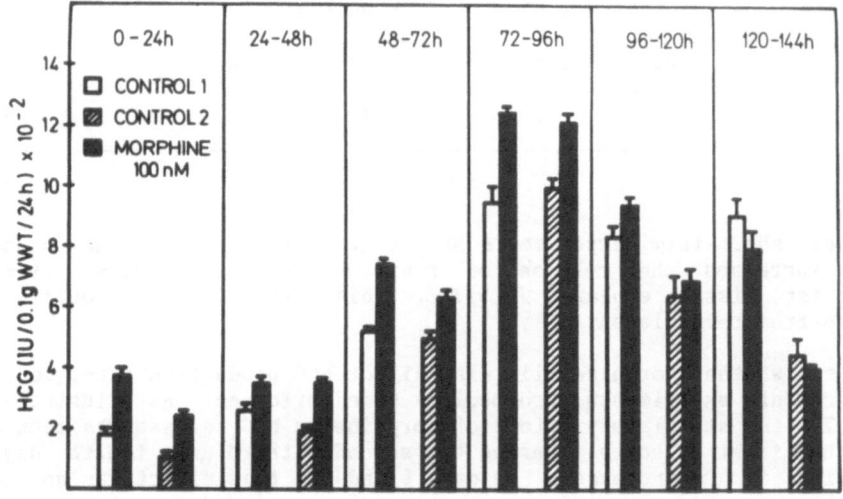

Figure 7.   Morphine effect on hCG production rate in first trimester placentae. Culture as in Figure 4. Results expressed as IU/0.1 g wwt/24 h. Each bar is the mean ± SEM from five independent cultures. Control 1 and 2 = controls from two individual placentae.

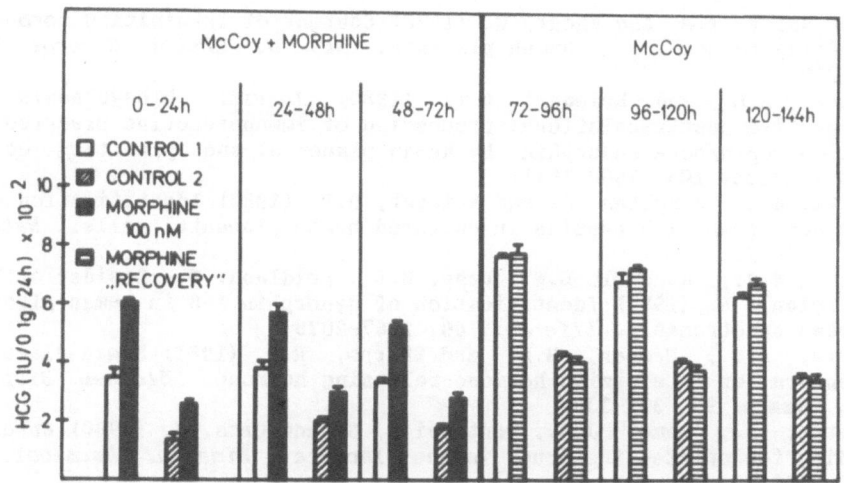

Figure 8. Reversibility of morphine effect on hCG production. Culture procedure as described for Figure 4. Results expressed as IU/0.1 g wwt/24 h. Each bar is the mean value ± SEM from five independent cultures. Control 1 and 2 = controls from two individual placentae.

these experiments falls within the range of Kd values for some opiates,[23] it is tempting to speculate that our results support a role for opiate peptides in the autocrine or paracrine[24] regulation of hCG synthesis and release by first trimester trophoblast.

These results confirm that trophoblast tissue explant technique can be used to study hCG synthesis and release and their regulation. The tissue retained its viability for up to six days in culture and responded selectively to exogenous stimulation. How relevant the *in vitro* results may be for *in vivo* situation, and how to evaluate them, remains to be elucidated.

REFERENCES

1. Belleville, F., Lasbenne, A., Nabet, P. and Paysant, P. (1978) HCS-HCG regulation in cultured placenta. *Acta Endocrinol.* **88**, 169-181.
2. Maruo, T., Matsuo, T., Ohtani, T., Hoshina, M. and Mochizuki, M. (1986) Differential modulation of chorionic gonadotropin (CG) subunit messenger ribonucleic acid levels and CG secretion by progesterone in normal placenta and choriocarcinoma cultured *in vitro*. *Endocrinology* **119**, 855-864.
3. Wilson, E.A., Jawad, M.J. and Dickson, L.R. (1980) Suppression of human chorionic gonadotropin by progestational steroids. *Am. J. Obstet. Gynecol.* **138**, 708-713.
4. Wilson, E.A., Jawad, M.J. and Powel, D.E. (1984) Effect of estradiol and progesterone on human chorionic gonadotropin secretion *in vitro*. *Am. J. Obstet. Gynecol.* **149**, 143-148.
5. Ho Yuen, B., Moon, Y.S. and Shin, D.H. (1986) Inhibition of human chorionic gonadotropin by prolactin from term human trophoblast. *Am. J. Obstet. Gynecol.* **154**, 336-340.
6. Gibbons, J.M., Mitnick, M. and Chieffo, V. (1975) *In vitro* biosynthesis of TSH- and LH-releasing factors by the human placenta. *Am. J. Obstet. Gynecol.* **121**, 127-131.

7. Siler-Khodr, T.M. and Khodr, G. (1978) Content of luteinizing hormone – releasing factor in the human placenta. *Am. J. Obstet. Gynecol.* **130**, 216–219.

8. Liotta, A.L. and Krieger, D.T. (1980) *In vitro* biosynthesis and comparative posttranslational processing of immunoreactive precursor of corticotropin/beta-endorphin by human placental and pituitary cells. *Endocrinology* **106**, 1504–1511.

9. Liotta, A.L., Houghten, R. and Krieger, D.T. (1982) Identification of a beta-endorphin-like peptide in cultured human placental cells. *Nature*, **295**, 593–595.

10. Ahmed, M.S., Randall, L.W., Dass, B.S., Fridland, G., Desiderio, D.M. and Tolun, E. (1987) Identification of dynorphin 1-8 in human placenta by mass spectrometry. *Life Sci.* **40**, 2067–2076.

11. Currie, A.J., Fraser, H.M. and Sharpe, R.M. (1981) Human placental receptors for luteinizing hormone-releasing hormone. *Biochem. Biophys. Res. Commun.* **99**, 332–338.

12. Valette, A., Reme, J.M., Pontonnier, G. and Cros, J. (1980) Specific binding for opiate-like drugs in the placenta. *Biochem. Pharmacol.* **29**, 2657–2661.

13. Ahmed, M.S., Byrne, W.L. and Klee, W.A. (1981) Solubilization of opiate receptors from human placenta. *Placenta* 3, 115–121.

14. Porthé, G., Valette, A. and Cros, J. (1981) Kappa-opiate binding sites in human placenta. *Biochem. Biophys. Res. Commun.* **101**, 1–6.

15. Belisle, S., Petit, A., Gallo-Payet, N., Bellabarba, D., Lehoux, J.G. and Lemaire, S. (1988) Functional opioid receptors in human placentas. *J. Clin. Endocrinol. Metab.* **66**, 283–289.

16. Khodr, G. and Siler-Khodr, T. (1978) The effect of luteinizing hormone-releasing factor on human chorionic gonadotropin secretion. *Fertil. Steril.* **30**, 301–314.

17. Siler-Khodr, T., Khodr, G., Valenzuela, G. and Rhode, J. (1986) Gonadotropin-releasing hormone effects on placental hormones during gestation: I. Alpha-human chorionic gonadotropin, human chorionic gonadotropin and human chorionic somatomammotropin. *Biol. Reprod.* **34**, 245–254.

18. Valette, A., Tafani, M., Porthé, G., Pontonnier, B. and Cros, J. (1983) Placental kappa opiate-binding sites: interaction with dynorphin and its possible implication in hCG secretion. *Life Sci.* **33**, 523–526.

19. Čemerikić, B., Genbačev, O., Šulović, V. and Beaconsfield, R. (1988) Effect of morphine on hCG release by first trimester human trophoblast *in vitro. Life Sci.* **42**, 1773–1779.

20. Petraglia, F., Sawchenko, P., Wlim, A.T., Rivier, J. and Vale, W. (1987) Localization, secretion and action of inhibin in human placenta. *Science* 237, 187–189.

21. Beaconsfield, R., Čemerikić, B., Genbačev, O. and Šulović, V. (1987) The placenta as a model for toxicity screening of new molecules. In: "Trophoblast Research". Editors: R.K. Miller and H.A. Thiede, Plenum Press, New York and London, pp 343–356.

22. Golander, A., Barrett, J.R., Tyrey, L., Fletcher, W.H. and Handwerger, S. (1978) Differential synthesis of human placental lactogen and human chorionic gonadotropin *in vitro. Endocrinology* **102**, 597–605.

23. Ahmed, M.S. and Cavinato, A.G. (1987) Partial purification of the opioid receptor from human placenta. In: "Trophoblast Research". Editors: R.K. Miller and H.A. Thiede, Plenum Press, New York and London, pp 279–287.

24. Petraglia, F., Fachineti, F., M'Futa, K., Ruspa, M., Bonavera, J.J., Gandolfi, F. and Genazzani, A.R. (1986) Endogenous opioid peptides in uterine fluid. *Fertil. Steril.* **46**, 247–251.

EFFECTS OF DECIDUAL PROLACTIN ON AMNIO-CHORION WATER PERMEABILITY

G.H. Mulder

Free University Hospital, Amsterdam, The Netherlands

Pregnancy in most mammals involves the exchange of gases with, the supply of nutrients to, and the removal of metabolic waste from the developing embryo or fetus in utero, through the intervention of the placenta. These "mechanical" functions of the placenta seem more or less known. However, the hormonal role of this organ is still a matter of much debate.

As well as placental transport and exchange of materials, there is another important source of interaction between mother and fetus: the amniotic fluid within its surrounding membranes - the amnion-chorion-decidua triad. Communication between fetus and mother through the amniotic fluid appears to be of a different nature from that through the placenta. While the amniotic fluid offers an indirect pathway by acting as a receptacle for fetal secretions from the urogenital, skin and lung systems, the placenta enables a much more direct exchange to take place between the maternal and fetal circulations. Consequently, placental interactions may well function on an acute, moment to moment basis, while the much slower interaction through amniotic fluid-amnion-chorion-decidua seems likely to preclude a rapid exchange of signals between the two organisms. In addition, the fetal end of the amniotic fluid communication channel is constituted by a derivative of the fetal circulation, rather than the circulation itself, as in the case of the placenta.

The nature and the amount of amniotic fluid seems to be important for the normal development of the human fetus. Conditions involving decreased or increased amounts of amniotic fluid often lead to, or are the consequence of, fetal or maternal pathology.[1-4] More often than not however, the exact mechanism behind abnormalities in amniotic fluid volume or composition is not known. Since the normal physiological process of amniotic fluid interaction between mother and fetus is also unknown, more information on this state of affairs is needed before pathological derangements can be studied with any success.

We are interested in the role the fetal membranes can play in determining amniotic fluid volume and composition. The other systems active in this respect are fetal swallowing, fetal urination, fetal lung fluid production, fetal skin exchange, and, possibly, umbilical cord exchange. Since there are technical and ethical considerations that make it unacceptable to study this *in vivo*, the only alternative is an *in vitro* study.

In a number of animal species prolactin (PRL) plays an important role in fluid and mineral balance. Examples of these are lactation in mammals and salt to fresh water transfer in certain fish.[5-9] An extensive review of the many possible roles of prolactin has been made.[10] When considering the possible role of prolactin during human pregnancy its extremely high levels in amniotic fluid are striking. Around the 20th week of pregnancy the concentration of prolactin in amniotic fluid is 1.5 to 2 orders of magnitude higher than in the maternal or fetal circulation. It is tempting to consider the presence of such large amounts of a peptide hormone in amniotic fluid (at a point in time when the fetal skin seems to have reached a state of relative impermeability) as an indicator of a physiological process.

We have asked two specific questions: first, is decidual prolactin production affected by osmolality changes in the incubation fluid and second, does decidually-produced prolactin affect the transfer of water and/or ions through fetal membranes?

The answer to both questions seems to be in the affirmative.

METHODS

Two methods were employed for studying the relationship between decidual prolactin and osmolality. In the first, designated method P, the objective was to monitor the production of prolactin by fetal membranes under conditions that permit both faces of the membrane to be exposed to fluids of the same or different nature, and where, in addition, frequent fluid sampling is possible. The second method, M, centred on the detection of mass transfer through fetal membranes under conditions where the local prolactin concentration can be modified, either by adding exogenous prolactin or by affecting endogenous prolactin secretion.

In method P fresh fetal membranes (2 x 2 cm) were loosely mounted between two vertical pieces of nylon netting having pores of approximately 0.5 mm in size. The nets were held taut by a flat square metal holder clamped between the two halves of a Plexiglass incubation chamber. The capacity of each chamber could be varied between 4 and 10 ml, and fluid introduced into or removed from each half through openings on either side or at the top. The build-up of unstirred layers close to the incubated membranes was prevented by the action of two magnetic stirring bars that could spin freely in small wells carved into the bottom plate of each half chamber. The assembled chamber was placed in a small glass water bath and kept at 37° C on a hot plate magnetic stirrer; the latter ensured fluid mixing in the chambers. The entire apparatus, which was constructed in duplicate, could be used for static incubations where each half of the chamber could be sampled manually, or dynamically by fluid being introduced continuously from the side of the compartments leaving the chambers through the openings at the top. A peristaltic pump and a fraction collector complete this automated addition and sampling arrangement. By using a four-channel pump and a four-channel fraction collector we could run two of these experiments simultaneously (Fig. 1).

In method M the objective was to measure mass transfer. After some experimentation we decided on the continuous mass measurement of the contents of a small compartment separated from outside fluid by fetal membranes. To that end, concentric Plexiglass cylinders were constructed with diameters of 14 and 18 mm respectively and a height of 6 cm. The space in between the cylinders was taken up by a coil of flexible, thin-walled silicon rubber tubing through which a mixture of 95% O_2 and 5% CO_2 was bubbled. The open, bottom end, of the cylinders could be sealed off with a

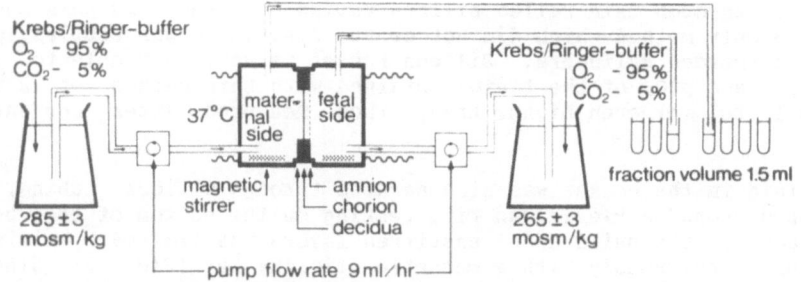

Figure 1.   Double-sided perifusion of mounted fetal membranes.

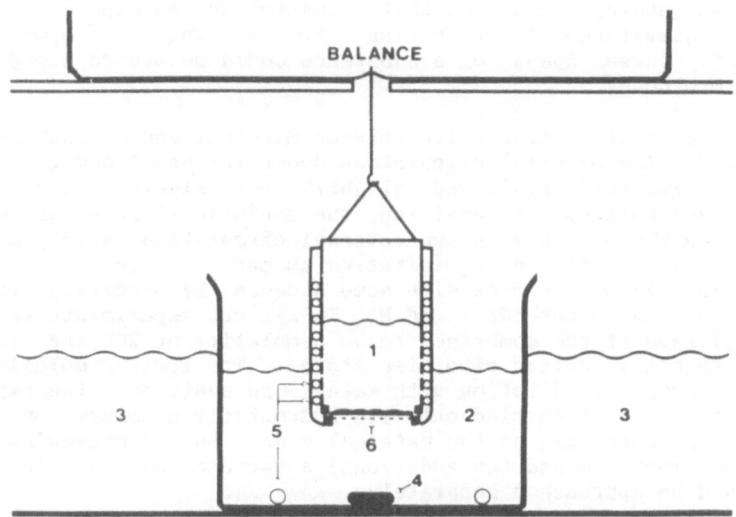

Figure 2.   Continuous weight monitoring of immersed incubation
             chamber - 1 small (usually fetal) compartment, 2-4ml; 2
             large (usually maternal compartment, 40 ml; 3 37° C
             water bath;   4 magnetic stirring bar; 5 silicon tubing
             for aeration; 6 nylon support net under membrane tissue.

ring on which a circular piece of fetal membrane could be fixed,   supported
by a nylon net. Through the open top end the cylinders could be filled with
(4 ml of) fluid and then placed in a beaker that could also be filled   with
fluid (40 ml).

    Using a metal wire of adjustable length the cylinders   were   suspended
from an electronic milligram balance (Mettler PE 360) placed on a   table
above the beaker. This balance senses the mass of an object without any
movement of the latter. Any potential movement of the weighing mechanism is
electronically compensated. This compensation is an electric current which
is read off as the mass. The advantage of this technique is that there is
no vertical movement by the cylinders inside the beakers, thereby obviating
the necessity for correcting weight changes through changes in submerged
volume.   Proper adjustment of the wire length allows the fluid level in the
cylinder to be placed anywhere from between 4 cm below to 4 cm above the
level in the beaker. Depending on which side of the membrane faces towards
the space in the cylinder or the space in the beaker, we could create
"fetal" and "maternal" compartments of between 4 and 40 ml (Fig. 2).

Aeration through thin-walled silicon tubing was used, as this appeared to be the only method which did not create disturbing gas bubbles on or under the submerged cylinders. Silicon rubber is very permeable to gases, and the pO_2 and pCO_2 of the fluids obtained with this method of aeration were equal to, or even higher than, those measured after conventional bubbling.

The fluid in the beaker was also aerated through silicon tubing, this time wrapped around a Plexiglass ring resting on the bottom of the beaker. As in method P, the build-up of unstirred layers was limited by mixing the fluid almost continuously with a magnetic stirring bar (Fig. 2). Since the apparent weight of the suspended cylinders was affected by fluid currents, the stirring action was halted 10 seconds before each recording and resumed 2 seconds after it had been made. The time intervals between each recording could be varied from 16 to 640 seconds. The entire apparatus was constructed in quadruplicate, so that a control and an experiment could be carried out simultaneously with tissue from one and the same patient. Alternatively, three doses of a substance could be tested along with a control or zero dose.

In vivo the fetal membranes lie between maternal endometrium and fetal amniotic fluid. The maternal circulation shows the usual osmotic value of 285 mosm/kg. Amniotic fluid is slightly but significantly lower in osmolality: 265 mosm/kg. In addition, the amniotic fluid pressure is 2 cm H_2O higher than the pressure in the maternal circulation. Attempts to mimic closely *in vivo* conditions by imitating as many as possible of these parameters *in vitro* can meet with some success by treating the fetal membranes according to methods P and M. In all our experiments we exposed the maternal face of the membranes to an osmolality of 285 and the fetal face to 265 mosm/kg, unless otherwise stated. The lower osmolalities were prepared by appropriate dilution with water. In addition, the experiments in method M were always carried out with hydrostatic pressures on the fetal side of 2 cm H_2O more than on the maternal side, unless otherwise stated. In these experiments we had the additional advantage that each face of the membrane could be approached separately.

We used fetal membranes from full term vaginal deliveries where pregnancy had been uncomplicated. No anaesthetics or other drugs were used before or during delivery. Immediately after delivery the placentae with adhering membranes were inspected for macroscopic abnormalities. If none were visible, the tissue was transferred to our laboratory in a suitable container as rapidly as possible. Care was taken to prevent cooling or drying of the tissue during handling.

Square pieces of membrane (3-10 cm²) were cut out not closer than 2 cm from the rim of the placenta. These pieces were then rinsed twice in Krebs-Ringer-bicarbonate-glucose at 37° C. The composition of this fluid is (ions in mMol): NaCl 119, KH_2PO_4 1.2, KCl 4.7, $MgSO_4$ 1.2, $CaCl_2$ 2.5, $NaHCO_3$ 24.9, glucose 11.1. To this, we added human serum albumin 2 mg/ml and streptomycin and gentamycin sulphate 0.1 and 0.5 mg/ml respectively. The pH was kept at 7.25 to 7.40 by the gas mixture.

The tissue was then mounted in the apparatus. The first 60 minutes of incubation or superfusion yielded widely varying results. This was probably the consequence of birth stresses and manipulation of the tissue. This initial 60 mn period was regarded as an equilibration period, during which few, if any, recordings were made.

In a number of experiments prolactin preparations from varying sources were used. Human and ovine pituitary prolactin were obtained from Dr. P.J. Lowry (National Institutes of Health, Bethesda Md, USA). Prolactin from amniotic fluid was prepared in our own laboratory by fractionated ammonium sulphate precipitation followed by fractionated ethanol precipitation, then repeated Sephacryl chromatography, locating the prolactin peaks by radio-immunoassay. Prolactin-enriched column fractions were obtained in the range of molecular weight of 22, 40 and 60 kD, possessing immunoactivities of 18, 76 and 40 U/g protein, taking one unit of prolactin to represent approximately 30 microgrammes of peptide. These prolactin fractions were designated as fractions 3, 2 and 1 respectively. Obviously these preparations are far from the desired degree of purity. However, they contained no measurable amounts of hPL, hCG, SP_1, AVP, OXY, LH or FSH, as assayed by various sensitive radioimmunoassays.

RESULTS

Method P

Experiments with this method can be divided into two groups: those where the signal (change in osmolality) was presented to the maternal face, and those where it was presented to the fetal face. The first test of the efficacy of the method was that the prolactin secretion from the decidual face was always higher than that of the fetal face. This indicated that there were no major leaks in the mounted membrane due to the concentration difference.

An osmolality increase from 285 to 325 mosm/kg effected by adding sucrose to the fluid circulating at the maternal face resulted in a rapid and strong transient increase in prolactin secretion from that maternal side (Fig. 3). Although the maternally-applied osmotic signal could not be detected in the fluid at the fetal side, this latter compartment also showed a transient increase in prolactin secretion - though of lesser magnitude and at a later point in time than the response at the maternal face (Fig. 4).

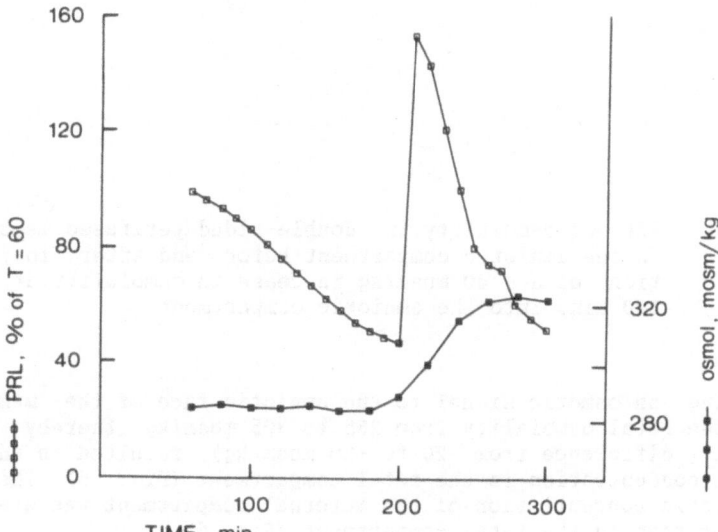

Figure 3.   PRL and osmolality in double-sided perifused membranes in the decidual compartment before and after introduction of a + 40 mosm/kg increase in osmolality at t = 160 min, into the decidual compartment.

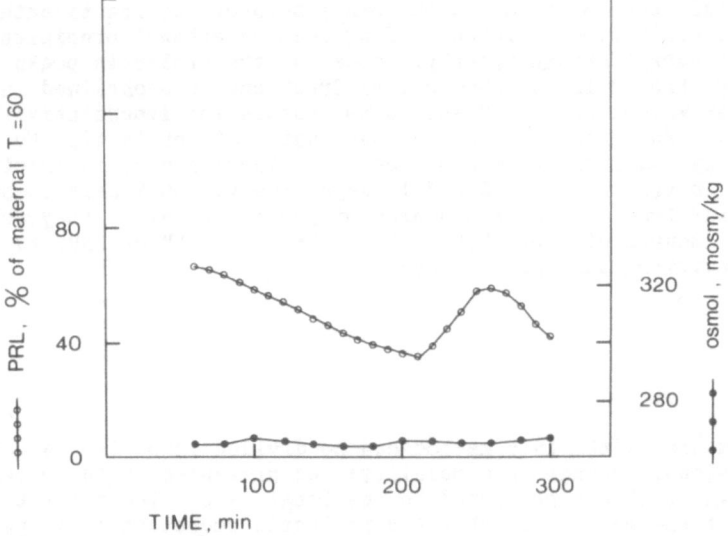

Figure 4.   PRL and osmolality in the amniotic compartment of the
experiment depicted in Fig. 3.

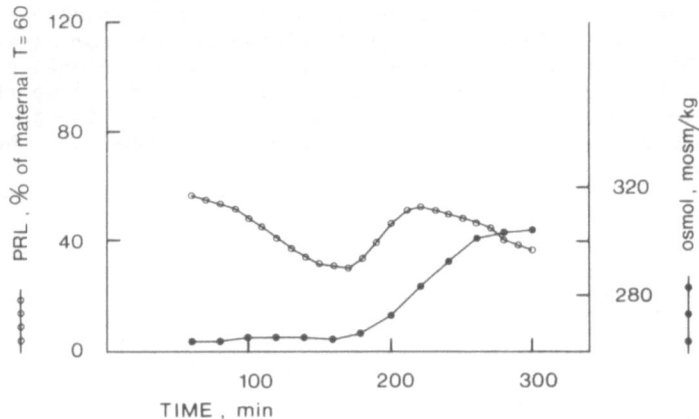

Figure 5.   PRL and osmolality in double-sided perifused membranes
in the amniotic compartment before and after introduction of a + 40 mosm/kg increase in osmolality at t =
160 min, into the amniotic compartment.

    Presenting an osmotic signal to the amniotic face of the membrane by
increasing the fetal osmolality from 265 to 305 mosm/kg (thereby reversing
the osmolality difference from −20 to +20 mosm/kg), resulted in an increase
in prolactin concentration in the fetal compartment (Fig. 5). The increase
in the prolactin concentration of the maternal compartment was greater and
started later than in the fetal compartment (Fig. 6).

Method M

    This system was first of all evaluated to verify the experimental
design. A gradual increase in apparent weight of the suspended cylinders

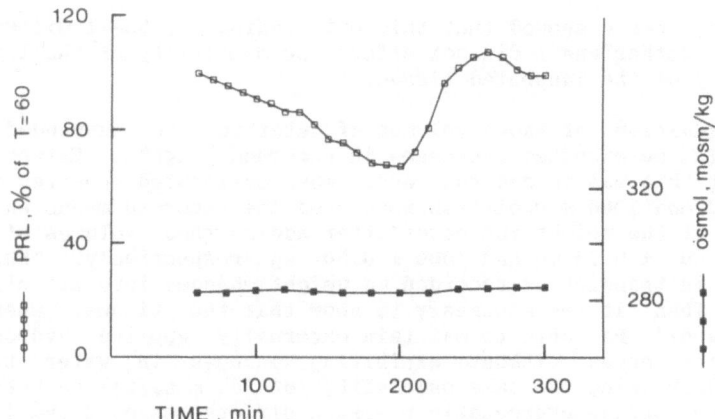

Figure 6.   PRL and osmolality in the decidual compartment of the
experiment depicted in Fig. 5.

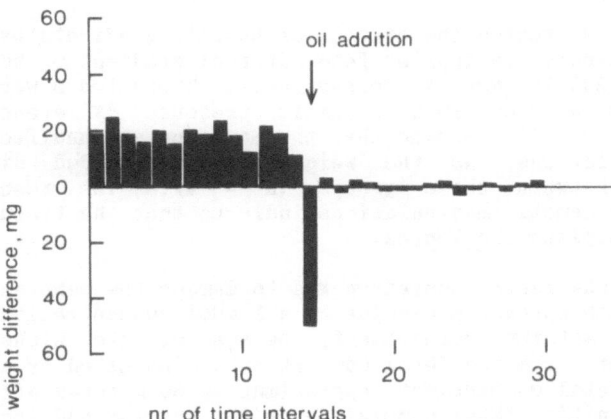

Figure 7.   Effect of adding oil onto the surface of the large
compartment of an immersed incubation chamber containing Parafilm. The differences in weight of successive
recordings have been plotted.

was noted, even if a piece of Parafilm was mounted in place of fetal
membrane. It became clear that this was due to a slow but steady
evaporation of the fluid in the outer bath (the beaker) which caused the
fluid level in that compartment to fall, thereby decreasing the submerged
volume of the cylinders, which increased the apparent weight of these
suspended objects. Since it is difficult to pinpoint deviations from a set
of data when the baseline shows an unsteady drift, the problem was tackled
by spreading a thin layer of oil on the surface of the liquid in the
beaker.

    Figure 7 shows the effects on the data when a cylinder, sealed off
with a piece of Parafilm instead of fetal membrane, is observed before and
after spreading oil on to the water surface of the outer bath. In this and
the following graphs the weight differences between two subsequent
recordings are depicted, rather than the weights themselves. Presenting the
data in such a manner made the findings much clearer and more concise, as
well as permitting better comparisons between various experiments.

Separate tests showed that this oil (Ondina 32, Shell Oil Company, The Hague, The Netherlands) did not affect the osmolality of the liquids, nor the vitality of the incubated tissue.

The addition of known volumes of water to the suspended cylinders should yield the expected increases in recorded weights. Extensive testing showed that this was indeed the case. When calibrated pipettes of volumes between 50 and 1000 microlitres were used the recorded means and standard deviations of the weight increases after adding these volumes of water (n = 20) were 50 ± 0.13 mg and 1000 ± 0.50 mg respectively. Thus we felt confident in translating recorded mg weight changes into microlitre water transfer. Then it was necessary to show that the tissue, when properly mounted, would be able to maintain externally applied hydrostatic and osmotic differences without exhibiting changes in water transfer or leakage. When using the same osmolality (of 285 mosm/kg) on both sides of the membrane applied hydrostatic pressure differences of 2 and 4 cm of H_2O, which by themselves would tend to drive fluid out of the inner, fetal compartment, did not cause a decrease of the weight of the cylinders, compared .with 0 cm H_2O pressure difference. This showed that correctly mounted tissue can actively withstand hydrostatic pressure differences of up to 4 cm of H_2O before starting to show signs of leakage.

Similarly, we tested the effects of osmotic gradients by increasing or decreasing the normally applied feto-maternal gradient of 265-285 mosm/kg to 265-305 and 285-285 mosm/kg respectively. These tests were carried out while applying a 2 cm H_2O hydrostatic pressure difference across the membrane. The results showed that the membrane was unaffected by these osmotic manipulations, as the weight changes recorded did not differ significantly between these groups (n = 4). The results of these hydrostatic and osmotic manipulations indicate that the tissue we used can withstand the applied challenges.

A further challenge undertaken was to damage the membrane expressly by poisoning it with potassium cyanide at a 1 mMol concentration. The effect was that the maternal compartment, because of its higher osmolality, attracted water from the fetal compartment, indicated by a decrease in weight of the fetal compartment. Approximately 60 minutes after introducing the KCN, the initial fetal osmolality of 265 mosm/kg had increased to 282 mosm/kg. This increase could not be explained completely by the measured amount of water transferred, indicating that there must have been some counter-transfer of ions towards the fetal compartment. The osmolality on the maternal side did not change significantly, probably because this compartment has a 10 times greater volume than the fetal one, which could mask possible effects on ion concentration.

The morphology of the incubated membranes as seen on light microscopy showed no obvious changes compared with unincubated tissue.

As a result of all the foregoing we felt confident our system could be used to study the effects of added substances on the permeability of human fetal membranes *in vitro*.

Pituitary prolactin whether of ovine or human origin, in concentrations of up to 5 µg/ml (ovine) or 0.5-1 µg/ml (human) did not produce any effects on either the amniotic or decidual side of the membranes. The only clear, consistent and repeatable effects were seen with human amniotic fluid prolactin, in concentrations of up to 1 µg/ml, added to the amniotic face of the membrane. Figures 8 and 9 show the effect of AF-PRL fraction 1 on amnion and decidua respectively, and Figures 10 and 11 the effects of AF-PRL fraction 2 on amnion and decidua. The specificity of these effects was illustrated by the finding that anti-PRL (raised against human

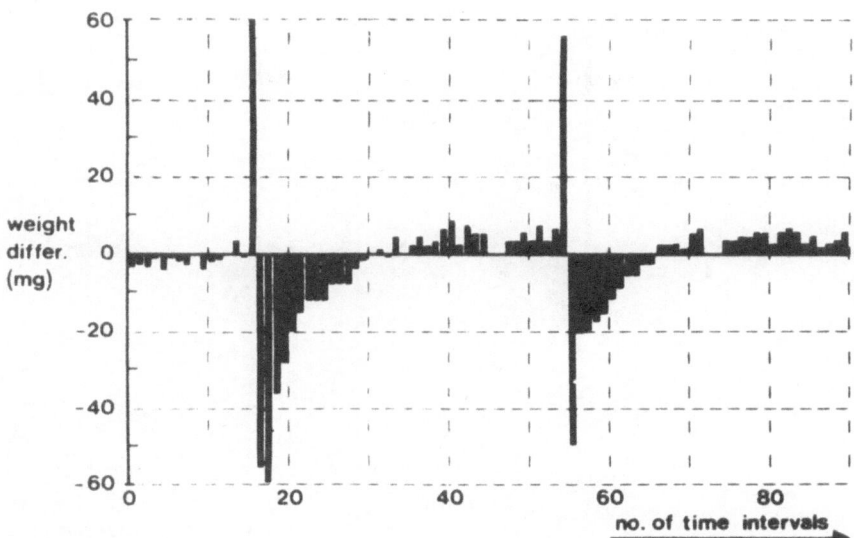

Figure 8. Effect of weight differences of an immersed incubation
chamber after introducing amniotic fluid PRL fraction 1
into the amniotic compartment at the 16th and 55th time
interval.

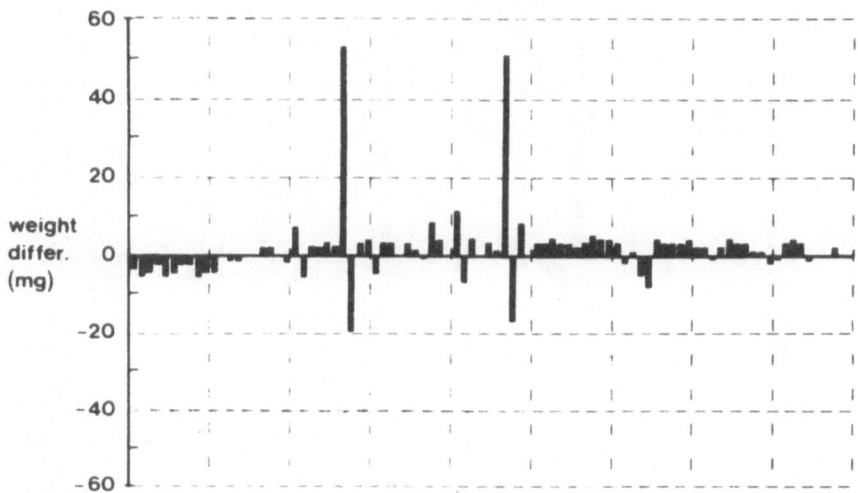

Figure 9. Effect of adding amniotic fluid PRL fraction 1 into the
decidual compartment of immersed incubation chambers,
at the 27th and 47th time interval.

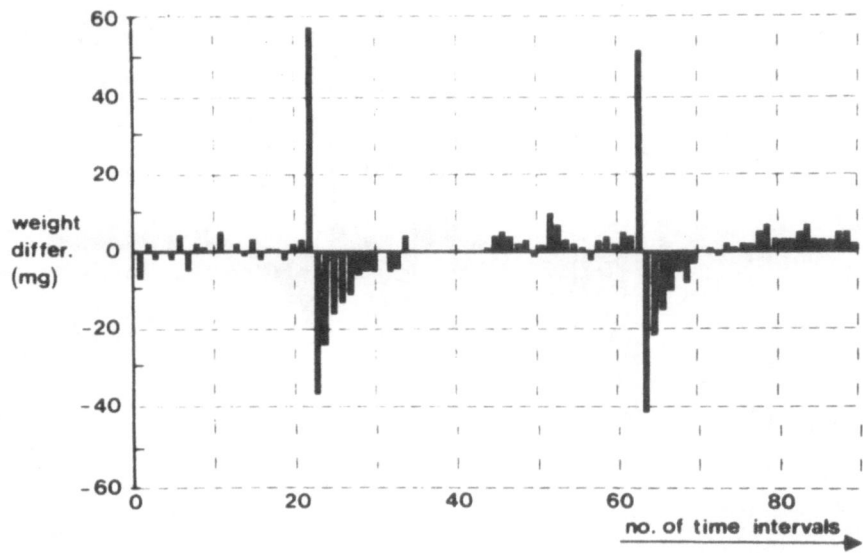

Figure 10. Effect of weight differences of an immersed incubation chamber after introducing amniotic fluid PRL fraction 2 into the amniotic compartment at the 23rd and 63rd time interval.

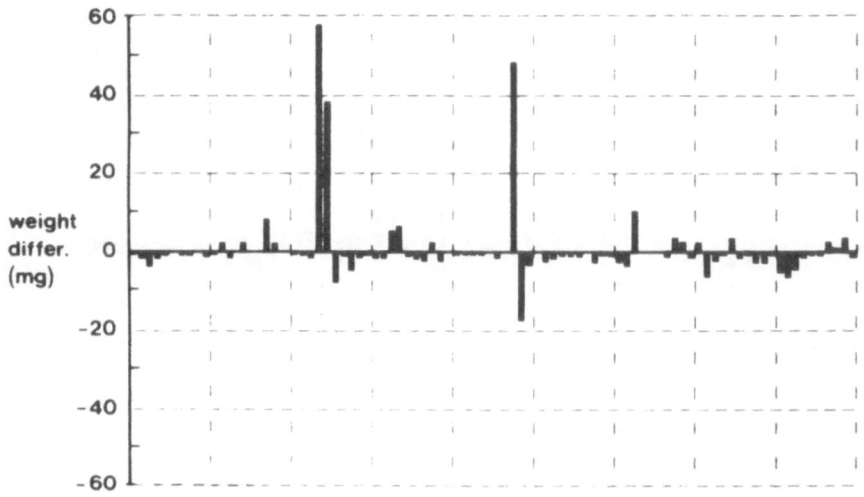

Figure 11. Effect of adding amniotic fluid PRL fraction 2 into the decidual compartment of immersed incubation chambers, at the 24th and 48th time interval.

pituitary PRL) was able to block the observed effects on amnion. The antiserum by itself was ineffective in changing water transfer.

DISCUSSION

The methods described above make it possible to study the relationship between decidual prolactin production and fetal membrane water/ion transfer.

From evaluation of our preparations it is evident that the membranes are alive and functioning. The fact that applied osmotic and hydrostatic gradients are maintained in the presence of a piece of semipermeable membrane indicates that some active mechanism prevents these gradients from disappearing. The fact that a metabolic poison renders the membranes "leaky" shows this active mechanism can be blocked. Decidually-produced prolactin is preferentially secreted into the maternal compartment, supporting data that point towards the decidua as the main source of amniotic fluid prolactin. So our system seems to function satisfactorily for experimentation.

Some of the results merit closer attention. Figures 3 and 4 (method P), show that a maternally applied osmotic signal induces a transient increase of prolactin secretion into both the maternal and fetal compartments. The rise in prolactin concentration in the fetal compartment occurs at a later point in time than in the maternal one. The question arises whether this increase of prolactin concentration in the fetal compartment is simply the result of prolactin diffusion, or transport from decidua through chorion and amnion into the extracellular space at the fetal face, or from amniotic prolactin secretion. The question becomes more intriguing when considering Figures 5 and 6. Here the signal was offered to the fetal face of the membrane. The results were a transient increase of prolactin secretion in both fetal and maternal compartments, but in this case the increase in the fetal compartment preceded the one in the maternal compartment. This finding seems to suggest that the amnion could be a possible source of amniotic fluid prolactin, since it seems unlikely that decidual prolactin could travel more quickly through chorion-amnion into the fetal compartment than through decidua into the maternal compartment.

An additional point has to be considered: the osmotic signal, applied to the fetal face, is not transmitted to the maternal compartment. Yet there is a clear response of the decidual tissue in terms of prolactin secretion. One explanation for this phenomenon could be the existence of cell-to-cell communication, where amnion cells can "sense" an osmotic change in their micro-environment, and can "signal" this change to the decidua, communicating through the chorion. Such an idea could be confirmed or rejected by using membranes before and after mechanical separation between amnion and chorion-decidua. Clearly a number of interesting questions remain to be answered.

In method M the apparent weight of a suspended, partly submerged, fluid-filled chamber is continuously measured. The fluid content of this chamber bears a direct relation to the recorded weight, in that additions of separate, known volumes of water to the volume of this object result in expected, precise levels of recorded weight increase. Although we have not provided proof that weight increases can be interpreted as volume increases we have nevertheless taken the data to represent such volume changes. One phenomenon could affect this reasoning: tissue swelling. This is unlikely to have occurred in our experiments as shown by the following considerations: When the fetal aspect points upwards toward the 4 ml compartment, suspended from the balance, the decidual face points toward the larger maternal compartment. If the tissue took up fluid from the stationary, maternal compartment, this would become evident by an increase of the apparent weight of the suspended fetal compartment. If on the other hand, tissue swelling were caused by fluid uptake from the fetal chamber, no change in recorded weight could have occurred. On occasion, we have noted some tissue oedema at the end of an experiment. This observation bore no relation to the recorded weight changes. Therefore it seems unlikely that the findings with method M result from processes other than water or ion transport through the fetal membranes.

One final comment should be made. As already stated, the preparations called AF-PRL 1 and AF-PRL 2 are impure. However, these preparations contained no activity of other hormones and were prepared according to prolactin immunoactivity data as a guideline. More importantly, the fact that the diuretic action of these preparations could be blocked by anti-PRL constitutes a strong argument in favour of the suggestion that the observed biological actions of "AF-PRL" are indeed the result of actions of amniotic fluid prolactin. In the face of evidence that prolactin from pituitary and prolactin from decidua are identical, we are obliged to consider posttranslational modifications (glycosylation and sialylation) as an explanation for the observed differences between the biological actions of human pituitary prolactin and human amniotic fluid prolactin.

REFERENCES

1. Jeffcoate, T.N.A. and Scott, J.S. (1959) Polyhydramnios and oligohydramnios. *Can. Med. Assoc. J.* **80**, 77-86.
2. Potter, E.L. (1965) Bilateral absence of ureters and kidney. A report of 50 cases. *J. Obst. Gyn. Brit. Cwlth.* **25**, 3-12.
3. Lingwood, B.E. and Wintour, E.M. (1983) Permeability of ovine amnion and amniochorion to urea and water. *Obstet. Gynecol.* **61**, 227-232.
4. Stangenberg, M., Vaclavincova, V. and Persson, B. (1982) Amniotic fluid volumes in pregnant diabetics during the last trimester. *Acta Obstet. Gynecol. Scand.* **61**, 313-316.
5. Lockett, M.F. and Nail, B.A. (1965) A comparative study of the renal actions of growth hormone and prolactin. *J. Physiol.* **180**, 147-156.
6. Chadwick, A. (1966) Prolactin-like activity in the pituitary glands of fishes and amphibians. *J. Endocrinol.* **35**, 75-81.
7. Mainoya, J.R. (1975a) Further studies on the action of prolactin on fluid and ion absorption by the rat jejunum. *Endocrinology* **96**, 1158-1164.
8. Mainoya, J.R. (1975b) Effects of bovine growth hormone, human placental lactogen and ovine prolactin on intestinal fluid and ion transport in the rat. *Endocrinology* **96**, 1165-1170.
9. Tyson, J.E. (1982) The evolutionary role of prolactin in mammalian osmoregulation: effects on fetoplacental hydromineral transport. *Semin. Perinatol.* **6**, 216-228.
10. Bern, H.A. and Nicoll, C.S. (1968) The comparative endocrinology of prolactin. *Recent Prog. Horm. Res.* **24**, 681-720.

EXTRACELLULAR MATRIX IN ENDOMETRIUM AND DECIDUA

John D. Aplin and Carolyn J.P. Jones

University of Manchester, England

Interstitial implantation places stringent requirements on the endome-trial environment. The extracellular matrix provides mechanical support for the epithelium, stroma, and vessels during the period of rapid cellular proliferation before ovulation. Subsequently, differentiative changes are initiated that prepare the tissue to accept an implanting embryo.[1] After implantation, a large population of trophoblast invades the decidua with the ultimate purpose of remodelling the maternal spiral arteries and increasing the flow of blood to the intervillous spaces.[2] These processes place new demands on the decidualising stromal matrix, which undergoes extensive reorganisation beginning at the peri-implantation period.[3] We have used immunochemical and ultrastructural approaches to examine hormone-dependent changes in the extracellular matrix of endometrial stroma in relation to the establishment of pregnancy.

Endometrial biopsies were collected at dilatation and curettage. Decidual biopsies were taken at termination of pregnancy. Tissue was either snap-frozen in liquid nitrogen (for light microscope immunocytochemistry) or fixed in 2.5% glutaraldehyde in 0.1 M sodium cacodylate buffer, pH 7.4 (for electron microscopy). Routine histopathological reports were consulted to confirm the date of the specimen and its normality.

For light microscopy, 6 µm cryosections were cut, air-dried and then stored at -15° C. Before staining, the sections were fixed in acetone for 3 minutes at ambient temperature. Details of the staining techniques have been published.[3] The antibodies to matrix components were as previously described with the additions of rabbit antibody to mouse entactin, which was a gift from Dr. B.L.M. Hogan,[4] monoclonal antibody GB3, which was raised to human amnion, and the two monoclonal anti-fibronectin antibodies IST-8 and IST-9 from Dr. L. Zardi.[5]

Tissue specimens for electron microscopy were cut into 1 mm cubes during fixation. These were post-fixed in 1% osmium tetroxide, dehydrated in graded alcohols and propylene oxide and embedded in Taab resin (Taab Laboratory Equipment Ltd., Reading, UK). Ultra thin sections were stained with uranyl acetate and lead citrate and examined in a Philips 301 electron microscope at 60 kV.

During the proliferative phase, the regenerating endometrial stroma produces a dense meshwork of collagen fibrils including collagen types I, III, V, and VI.[3,6] Figure 1a shows the distribution of type VI collagen in the proliferative phase. Fibronectin is also present (Fig. 1b) and some of the molecules contain the EDA segment recognised by monoclonal antibody IST-9 (Fig. 1c[5]). Staining with antibody IST-8, which recognises an epitope within the EDB domain, is very weak (Fig. 1d).

Early secretory phase stromal cells are often tightly packed, and the intercellular spaces can be seen to contain a meshwork of parallel fibrils (Fig. 2) of uniform diameter (28–33 nm). Fine fibrillar material is also visible, frequently intersecting the thicker fibrils at angles close to 90° (Fig. 3a). Deep, narrow recesses containing single fibrils are observed in

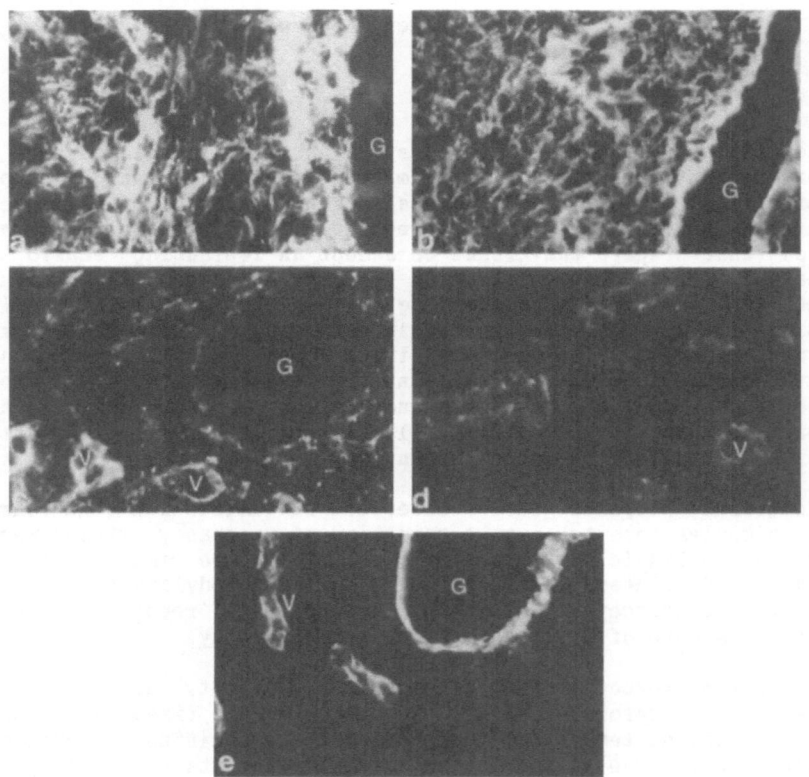

Figure 1.   Immunofluorescence of extracellular matrix components in proliferative phase endometrium. a: antibody to collagen type VI demonstrates an abundant network of stromal fibrils. b: polyclonal antibody to plasma fibronectin stains a tightly packed fibrillar array occupying the intercellular spaces in the stroma. c: anti-fibronectin monoclonal antibody IST-9 binds to blood vessel walls as well as a sparse array of interstitial fibrils. d: anti-fibronectin monoclonal antibody IST-8 shows a faint reactivity with vessel walls. e: staining with antibody to heparan sulphate proteoglycan reveals the glandular and vascular basement membranes. (x 400); G, gland; V, blood vessel.

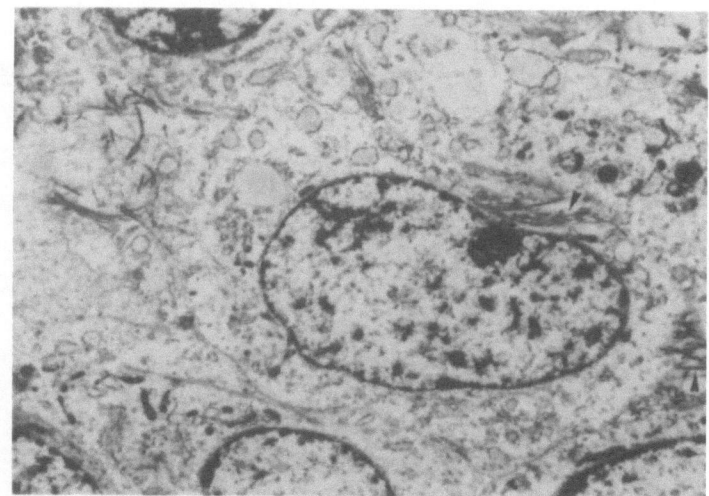

Figure 2.   Early secretory phase stroma showing tightly packed
cells with collagen fibrils and fibril bundles
(arrowhead) occupying the intercellular spaces. Note
the uniformity of diameter (approximately 30 nm) of the
fibrils (x 7500).

the stromal cells (Fig. 3a). Some cells show broad surface recesses in
which fibril bundles terminate abruptly at the plasma membrane (Fig. 3a),
suggesting sites of fibrillogenesis or lateral aggregation.[7] The stromal
cell cytoplasm contains prominent mitochondria, ribosomes, and rough
endoplasmic reticulum,[8,9] as well as Golgi apparatus and vesicles, all of
which is consistent with active matrix biosynthesis.

When proliferative phase tissue is stained with antibodies to the major
basement membrane components type IV collagen, laminin, and heparan
sulphate proteoglycan, a pattern of reactivity is observed in which binding
occurs to the glandular and luminal basement membranes (Fig. 1e).

In transmission electron microscopy (TEM) the glandular basal lamina
is, in some areas, resolved into a lamina densa about 30 nm thick and a
thinner lamina lucida (Fig. 3b). The matrix material immediately beneath
the glandular basal lamina is somewhat heterogeneous in appearance; in some
regions it contains bundles of banded fibrils approximately 30 nm in
diameter that resemble those seen in the deeper stroma (Figs. 3a; cf Fig.
2). In other areas (Fig. 3b) finer fibrils and amorphous deposits
predominate. Anchoring fibrils are present (Fig. 3b) and striated 30 nm
fibrils can be observed, appearing to terminate at the stromal side of the
glandular lamina densa (Fig. 3a).

MID SECRETORY PHASE ENDOMETRIUM

In the mid secretory phase, there are indications of matrix remodelling. The most sensitive index of this and subsequent changes in the
fibrillar matrix is the distribution of type VI collagen. In the proliferative phase, anti-collagen VI antibody reveals a uniform fibrillar array in
the stroma (Fig. 1a); in mid secretory phase most areas of the stroma are
still rich in type VI (Fig. 4a), but a degree of condensation into shorter
thicker fibrils and specks is evident, especially in the stroma away from
glands. In a few areas, a gradient of concentration is evident, the
periglandular stroma being rich in collagen VI while a diminution in
staining is apparent in deeper regions. However, the distribution of

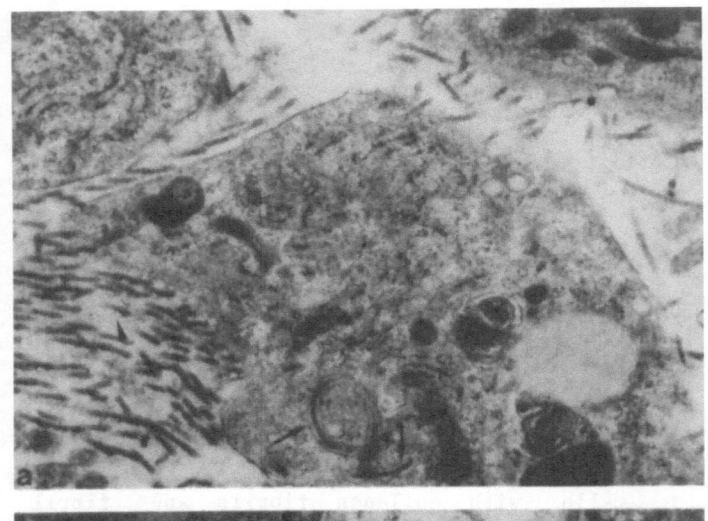

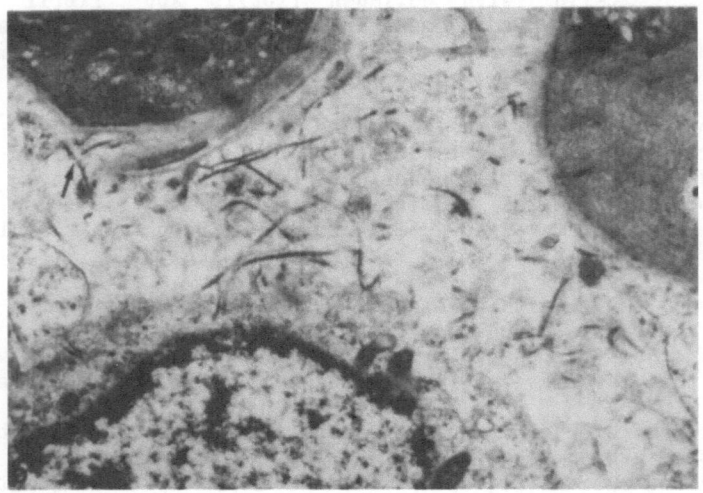

Figure 3.　TEM of early secretory phase periglandular stroma. a: cell showing two types of association with collagen fibrils: deep, narrow membrane-bounded recesses are evident within the cytoplasm (arrows); it is not clear whether or not these are contiguous with the cell surface. In addition there is a broad, shallow recess in the cell surface where fibrils in a bundle are closely apposed to the plasma membrane. Several fibrils are seen to terminate at the glandular basement membrane (asterisk). Fine fibrillar material (arrowhead) can be seen in association with the collagen (x 38000). b: In this area, sparse collagen fibrils and amorphous material predominate; glandular basement membrane can be seen with lamina lucida and lamina densa and, beneath the latter, occasional anchoring fibrils (arrow). The dating of the tissue is confirmed by the presence of a subnuclear glycogen deposit in a gland cell (asterisk, extreme right) (x 22750).

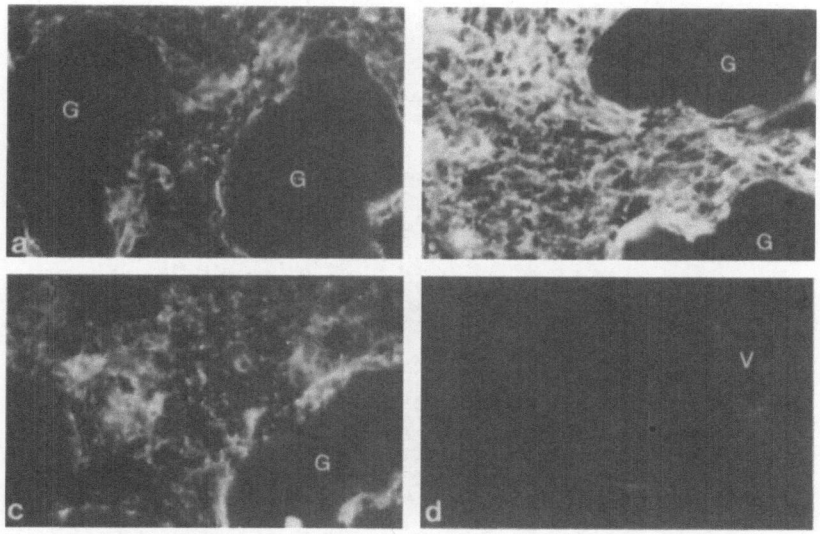

Figure 4. Immunofluorescence of matrix components in mid secretory phase endometrium. a: anti-collagen VI reveals a
partially fibrillar, partially punctuate distribution
of antigen with a generally reduced intensity compared
to that observed in the proliferative phase (cf. Fig.
1a). b: polyclonal anti-fibronectin stains intensely
throughout the stroma. c: monoclonal anti-fibronectin
antibody IST-9 stains the stroma more weakly than the
polyclonal antibody. d: little staining is observed
with monoclonal anti-fibronectin antibody IST-8 (x 400).

collagen VI in most areas still resembles that seen in the proliferative
phase, and reductions in staining intensity are much more apparent in late
secretory phase endometrium.[3] Blood vessel walls contain high concentrations of collagen VI in tissue from all parts of the secretory phase. In
contrast to collagen VI, fibronectin is abundant throughout the secretory
phase stroma and is detected with both polyclonal antibodies and monoclonal
antibody IST-9 (Figs. 4b,c). Antibody IST-8, in contrast, gives very poor
staining (Fig. 4d). Collagens III and V (and, presumably collagen I) are
abundant.[3]

FIRST TRIMESTER DECIDUA

In comparing extracellular matrix of first trimester decidua with that
of pre-implantation endometrium, several important changes are evident at
the ultrastructural level: a general reduction in fibril density (Fig. 5a),
though this is less obvious in the compacta; greater heterogeneity of
fibril diameters in decidual stroma (Fig. 5b) with fibrils (15-35 nm) often
being associated with fine fibrillar material (Fig. 5b); and a relative
infrequency of fibril bundles (Figs. 5a,b). Macrophages are often found in
close association with residual fibril bundles (Fig. 6).

Immunofluorescent staining with antibodies to collagens I, III, and V
demonstrates that all three are present in intercellular spaces, but the
reduced intensity of staining is consistent with a diminished fibril
density.[3] The molecular organisation is also altered, since type V collagen
epitopes are accessible to the antibody. This is in contrast to the
situation in endometrial stroma where collagen V is masked, probably by
copolymerisation with collagens I and III. Fibronectin is a prominent

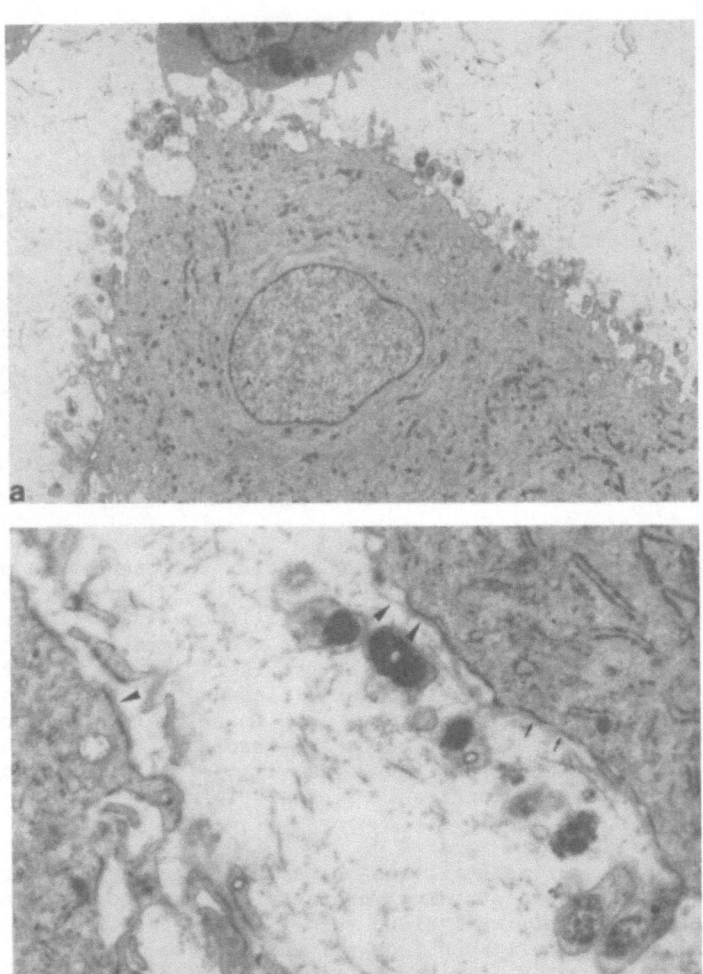

Figure 5. TEM of decidual stroma of late first trimester. a: low
          power view (x 7000) showing the general reduction in
          fibril density of the decidual extracellular matrix
          compared to early secretory endometrium (cf. Figs. 2,
          3). The complex surface architecture of a typical
          decidual cell is shown. The cell is in close contact
          with a mononuclear cell. b : heterogeneity of fibril
          diameter (15 - 35 nm) is evident, with little bundle
          formation. At this magnification (x 24500) the presence
          of a pericellular basal lamina is revealed (arrowhead).
          There is variation in its thickness (arrows) and
          cellular processes containing secretory material pro-
          trude through it (asterisks).

component in decidua and can be detected both with polyclonal antibodies
and with monoclonal antibody IST-9 (Fig. 7c), which establishes the
presence of molecular variants containing the EDA domain. None of the
fibronectin molecular variant containing the EDB domain is apparent, as
demonstrated by the absence of staining with the IST-8 antibody (Fig. 7d).
Decidual cells display cytoplasmic characteristics consistent with active

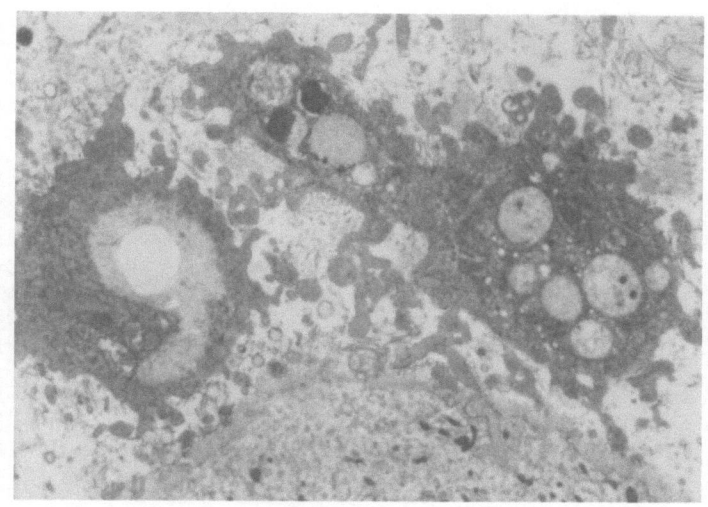

Figure 6.   Macrophages in intimate association with residual collagen bundles are also seen to make close contact with
a decidual cell (x 9000).

biosynthesis and have been shown to continue the production of collagens I,
III and V as well as fibronectin in the first trimester.[10]

An unexpected and interesting feature of decidualisation is the
appearance of a capsular basal lamina surrounding each cell.   By
immunofluorescence this can be shown to contain collagen IV, laminin and
heparan sulphate proteoglycan (Fig. 7a), but entactin has not been
detected[11] nor the epitope recognised by monoclonal antibody GB3.[12]
Monoclonal antibody G71, which also binds to an epitope present in many
human basement membranes[13] is weakly expressed by decidual cells, but some
of the staining appears to be cytoplasmic (not shown). Thus the decidual
cell elaborates a basal lamina that contains the three major structural
components, but not certain other molecules that occur beneath epithelial
cells.

The   presence of a basal lamina is confirmed by TEM and consists of a
pericellular structure which is absent from cells of the bone marrow-
derived population (Figs. 5a,b; 6). However, macrophages found in association with decidual cells frequently extend processes to make contact with
the lamina or even with the decidual cell surface (Fig. 6).   Some decidual
cells have an incomplete lamina, and considerable variations in its
thickness occur in individual cells (Fig. 5b) with occasional examples of
multilayering of the lamina (Fig. 8a). Even when complete, the lamina is
not a continuous structure, being punctuated by gaps through which protrude
small cellular processes (Figs. 5a,b). The latter often contain secretory
bodies (Fig. 5b). In areas of sparsely distributed decidual cells set in a
loose matrix of fibrils and ground substance, the basal laminae are
correspondingly associated with fewer fibrils. Some such areas contain an
abundant flocculent amorphous component (Fig. 8a) while in regions containing closely packed sheets of enlarged, differentiated decidual cells,
intercellular fibrillar "stitching" is often present. Here fibrils run
perpendicularly into the pericellular basal laminae, which thus appear to
play an organsing role (Fig. 8b).

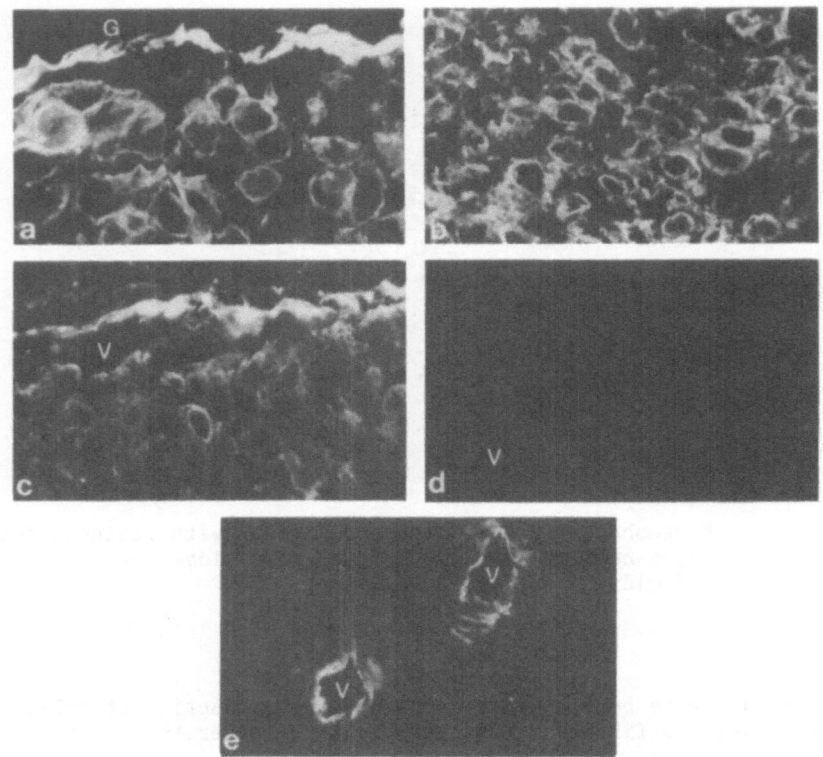

Figure 7. Immunofluorescence of matrix components in first trimester decidua. a: anti-heparan sulphate proteoglycan
binds to glandular basement membranes and also to the
pericellular matrices of enlarged decidual stromal
cells giving the appearance of an 'aura'. b: polyclonal
anti-fibronectin antibody binds in the pericellular
zones of decidual cells as well as being present in
some intercellular spaces. c: antibody IST-9 reacts
with some vessels and capillary spaces and weakly with
some decidual cell matrices. d: the IST-8 epitope is
absent from decidual tissue including blood vessels. e:
type VI collagen is also largely absent except for
blood vessel walls. This is in marked contrast to the
situation in proliferative endometrium (Fig. 1a) (x
400).

DISCUSSION

Previous TEM studies of human endometrial and decidual stroma[8,9,14-16]
concentrated more on cellular morphology than extracellular matrix, and
were performed without the benefit of compositional information on the
matrix. This information is now emerging as a result of the availability of
specific antibody probes.[3,10] The present study is an attempt to combine
these two approaches in order to characterise the hormonally dependent
processes of matrix remodelling, and predict the possible role of
extracellular matrix in the promotion and control of trophoblast invasion.

Stromal cells of the pre-implantation endometrium have previously been
thought[8] to be active in the elaboration of fibrillar collagens, and the
present results are fully consistent with this view. Trelstad and coworkers

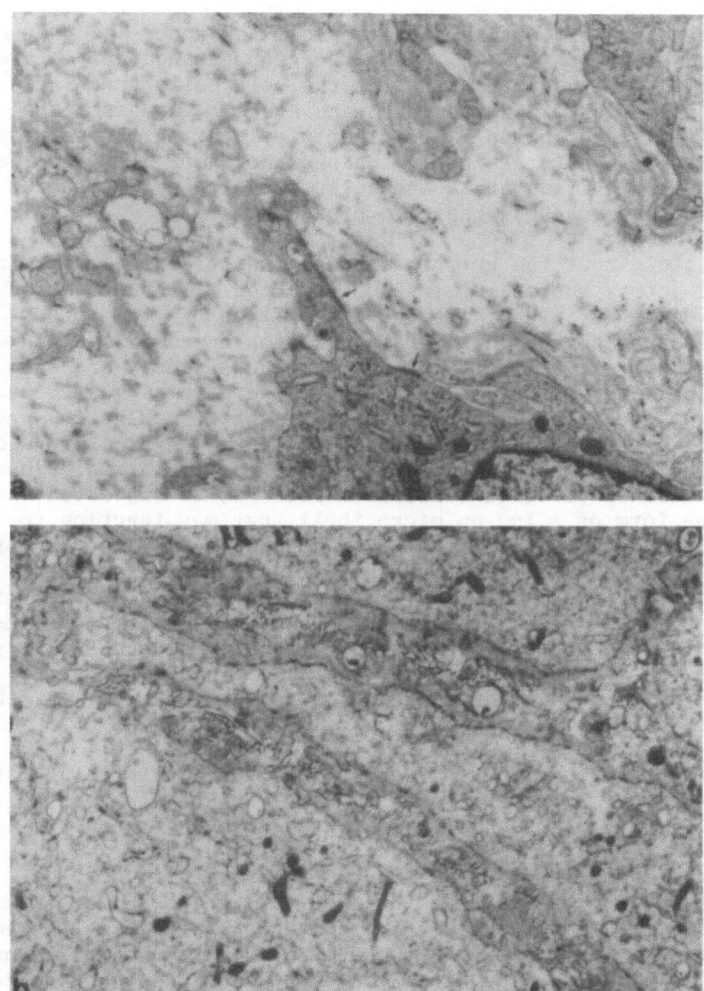

Figure 8.   TEM of late first trimester decidua. a: the pericellular basal lamina is multilaminar in places (asterisk)
and shows variation in thickness, with occasional
linear densities on the plasma membrane of the decidual
cell (arrows). In this area of the extracellular
matrix collagen fibrils are very sparse but there is an
abundant amorphous component (x 14200).   b: where
decidual cells are found in a more close packed array,
intercellular collagen fibrils produce a "stitching"
effect as they run perpendicularly into the pericellular basal laminas (x 12000).

have suggested that collagen fibrillogenesis in chick tendon occurs within
deep recesses in the fibroblast surface into which procollagen aggregates
are discharged before being added to the end of the growing fibril.[7,17]
However, narrow recesses containing single fibrils have been associated in
other tissues, especially gingiva and periodontal ligament, with internalisation and breakdown of fibrils.[18-20] In this case the recesses are

eventually pinched off within the cytoplasm to become phagolysosomes. In the Trelstad model of tendon, deep recesses subsequently fuse to form broader bundle-forming compartments at the cell periphery. These features – both deep fibril-containing recesses and broader compartments containing parallel fibril aggregates – are clearly evident in the early secretory phase endometrial stromal cell, and further work will be required to discover whether at this stage the cells are already degrading collagen; the evidence is strong that they are producing it.

It is likely that the uniform fibrils thus generated contain collagen type I, but ultrastructural immunolocalisation will be required to confirm this point and to investigate the disposition of the other collagens. Recent evidence obtained in several different human tissues suggests that copolymerisation of collagens I and III occurs widely and can result in fibrils with a wide variety of diameters.[21] We have suggested that collagen V is closely associated with other matrix macromolecules in endometrium.[3] It will be of particular interest to discover the physical form of collagen VI in endometrium, since little is known of this in normal tissues. On the basis of studies in placental villous stroma, it is suggested that collagen VI takes the form of a 100 nm microfibril that may function to cross-link the larger banded fibrils of the major collagens.[22] Thus the presence in endometrium of fine fibrillar material in association with the major fibrils is of interest. However, it is also noteworthy that in tendon, proteoglycans have been shown to bind to specific sites on the collagen fibril.[23] Studies are now required on glycosaminoglycan and proteoglycan distribution in endometrial stroma, especially in view of the report of increased hyaluronate production in mouse endometrium on the day of implantation.[24]

Ultrastructural examination of the decidual interstitial matrix during the first trimester reveals several features which, when comparison is made with the pre-implantation endometrium, suggest that extensive remodelling has occurred. There are reductions in fibril density and the number of fibril bundles, and an increase in the heterogeneity of fibril diameter. Taken together with the evidence that decidual cells produce and secrete a large variety of macromolecules[25] including collagens I, III and V,[10] this indicates that the remodelling process must involve a combination of matrix breakdown and de novo production. Macrophages, which are widespread in decidua,[26] are often found in association with decidual cells and have been shown to produce a procollagenase that resembles closely the one produced by human skin fibroblasts.[27] Activated macrophages have been shown to digest extracellular matrix components.[28] Morphological evidence of the involvement of macrophages in the breakdown of fibrillar collagen has also been obtained.[29] Thus it is reasonable to propose a role for these cells in the remodelling of the endometrial stroma. However, many other cell types also show collagenolytic activity[30] and some evidence is available that endometrial stromal cells may be involved in the breakdown as well as the elaboration of fibrillar matrix. Lysosome-like vesicles that contained fibrils in late secretory phase (predecidualising) stromal cells have been reported,[8] and similar features have been observed in the stromal cells of both mouse[31] and rat endometrium.[32] Functional tests on decidual stromal cells and macrophages would throw light on this matter.

Fibronectin is abundant in the endometrial interstitium throughout the period under study, though it may be anticipated that quantitative changes and physical re-organisation occur. Fibronectin is apparently retained in extracellular matrices by virtue of its binding to the collagens, fibrin, or glycosaminoglycans[33] and changes in their distribution must be expected to affect fibronectin. One important aspect of the analysis of fibronectin synthesis and deposition in a changing hormonal environment is to examine the pattern of differential splicing of mRNA that allows a single gene to give rise to several different polypeptide variants, the proportions of which vary between cell types.[5,34,35] The present study utilised two relevant monoclonal antibodies: IST-9, which binds to an epitope localised in the EDA domain[5] and IST-8, which binds to the EDB domain (G. Paolella, personal communication). The results suggest that most endometrial fibronectin lacks both of these domains. Staining in the vicinity of blood vessels with IST-9 and to a lesser extent IST-8 may indicate the production of some EDA- and EDB-positive fibronectin by endothelial cells in proliferative phase endometrium. There is also a small amount of IST-9 (but not IST-8) staining in the stroma in both endometrium and decidua. These results are not quantitative and do not allow estimates to be made of the relative proportions of the different variants. However, they do not support the idea that major differences occur in splicing patterns in endometrium and decidua as has been suggested.[35] These workers used different antibodies, but the reason for the discrepancy is not clear. Our results are in agreement with their finding[3] that adult capillary endothelial cells produce a fibronectin species containing the EDA domain.

The data presented here suggest that the decidual pericellular basal lamina, a structure that was observed initially in TEM by Wynn[14] and subsequently by several other groups,[3,10,36,37] contains collagen IV, laminin and heparan sulphate proteoglycan but not entactin[11] nor the epitope recognised by monoclonal antibody GB3.[12] The function of the basal lamina is an interesting matter for speculation. Its observed interaction with macrophages and mononuclear cells may suggest that it acts as a substratum for cell-cell or cell-matrix interaction. Its specific composition probably renders it resistant to the proteases involved in breakdown of interstitial matrix components. Interstitial fibrils are observed to terminate in the lamina, which may therefore act to organise or stabilise the sparser matrix of decidua and to immobilise the decidual cells themselves, which thus act to provide the matrix and cellular environment within which maternofetal interactions occur. It is also possible that it may act as a reservoir of immobilised growth factor for trophoblast or immune cells; binding of growth factors to matrix components has been observed in several other systems[38] and decidual cells are known to secrete growth factors. It is also relevant that mouse endometrial epithelial cells produce the growth factor CSF-1 which stimulates the proliferation and differentiation of mononuclear phagocytes.[39] It seems likely that decidual cells secrete various polypeptide products across the lamina by means of cytoplasmic processes which protrude through the lamina and contain secretory bodies. Thus this basal lamina does not act as a barrier to the diffusion of macromolecules.

In this study, changes are documented in the composition and ultrastructure of endometrial extracellular matrix during the menstrual cycle and in the first trimester of pregnancy; the most striking alterations are the reduction in fibril density, the appearance of the decidual pericellular basal lamina and the disappearance of interstitial collagen VI. It is clear that much more detailed work remains to be done on the precise dating of these changes, since the present study relied on histological dating of endometrium, the limitations of which have been demonstrated.[40] We have also been restricted to the study of decidua obtained in late first trimester only. However, the significance of these changes for implantation and early embryogenesis (including trophoblast invasion) may be considerable. We have suggested[3] that the specific loss of collagen VI, which may provide interfibrillar cross-links and the general reduction in fibril density may allow spaces or channels to become available in the tissue into which trophoblast migration may occur. We have also examined the interaction of the trophoblast-derived cell line BeWo with components of the decidual matrix and found that, of the components tested, fibronectin is the most efficient in promoting adhesion and shape change. These are obvious prerequisites of any cellular migratory activity. The presence in decidual matrix of fibronectin, which has been widely associated with matrix-modulated adhesion and migration,[33] is consistent with the idea that it may act as an anchorage molecule for migrating trophoblast. The changes described lend no support to the hypothesis that decidualisation contributes to maternal restriction of the invasion of trophoblast; on the contrary, all our observations suggest that decidualisation is a maternal process of preparation to accept invading trophoblast.

REFERENCES

1. Aplin, J.D. (1989) Cellular biochemistry of the endometrium. In: "Biology of the Uterus". Editors: R.M. Wynn and W.P. Jollie. Plenum, New York. In press.
2. Pijnenborg, R., Dixon G., Robertson, W.B. and Brosens, I. (1980) Trophoblastic invasion of human decidua from 8 to 18 weeks of pregnancy. *Placenta* 1, 3-19.
3. Aplin, J.D., Charlton, A.K. and Ayad, S. (1988) An immunohistochemical study of human endometrial extracellular matrix during the menstrual cycle and first trimester of pregnancy. *Cell Tissue Res.* 253, 231-240.
4. Cooper, A.R., Kurkinen, M., Taylor, A. and Hogan, B.L.M. (1981) Studies on the biosynthesis of laminin by murine parietal endoderm cells. *Eur. J. Biochem.* 119, 189-197.
5. Borsi, L., Carnemolla, B., Castellani, P., Rosellini, C., Vecchio, D., Allemanni, G., Chang, S.E., Taylor-Papadimitriou, J., Pande, H. and Zardi, L. (1987) Monoclonal antibodies in the analysis of fibronectin isoforms generated by alternative splicing of mRNA precursors in normal and transformed human cells. *J. Cell Biol.* 104, 595-600.
6. Dallenbach-HGellweg, G. (1981) "Histopathology of the endometrium". Springer-Verlag, Berlin.
7. Birk, D.E. and Trelstad, R.L. (1986) Extracellular compartments in tendon morphogenesis: collagen fibril, bundle and microaggregate formation. *J. Cell Biol.* 103, 231-240.
8. Wienke, E.C., Filiberto Calvazos, B.S., Hall, D.S. and Lucas, L.V. (1968) Ultrastructure of the endometrial stromal cell during the menstrual cycle. *Am. J. Obstet. Gynecol.* 102, 65-77.
9. More, I.A.R., Armstrong, E.M., Carty, M. and McSeveney, D. (1974) Cyclical changes in the ultrastructure of the normal endometrial stromal cell. *Brit. J. Obstet. Gynaecol.* 81, 337-347.
10. Kisalus, L.L., Herr, J.C. and Little, C.D. (1987) Immunolocalisation of extracellular matrix proteins and collagen synthesis in first trimester human decidua. *Anat. Rec.* 218, 402-415.
11. Carlin, B., Jaffe, R., Bender, B. and Chung, A.E. (1981) Entactin, a novel basal lamina-associated sulphated glycoprotein. *J. Biol. Chem.* 256, 5209-5214.
12. Verrando, P., Hsi, B-L., Yeh, C-J., Pisani, A., Serieys, N. and Ortonne, J-P. (1987) Monoclonal antibody GB3. A new probe for the study of human basement membranes and hemidesmosomes. *Exp. Cell Res.* 170, 116-128.
13. Aplin, J.D. and Seif, M.W. (1985) Basally located epithelial cell surface component identified by a novel monoclonal antibody technique. *Exp. Cell Res.* 160, 550-555.
14. Wynn, R.M. (1974) Ultrastructural development of the human decidua. *Am. J. Obstet. Gynecol.* 118, 652-670.
15. Wynn, R.M. (1977) Histology and ultrastructure of the human endometrium. In: "Biology of the Uterus". Editor: R.M. Wynn, Plenum, New York, pp 341-376.
16. Cornillie, F.J., Lauweryns, J.M. and Brosens, I.A. (1985) Normal human endometrium. An ultrastructural survey. *Gynecol. Obstet. Invest.* 20, 113-129.

17. Trelstad, R.L. and Silver, F.H. (1981) Matrix assembly. In: "Cell Biology of the Extracellular Matrix". Editor: E.D. Hay, Plenum, New York, pp 179-215.

18. Ten Cate, A.R. and Deporter, D.A. (1975) The degradative role of the fibroblast in the remodelling and turnover of collagen in soft connective tissue. *Anat. Rec.* 182, 1-14.

19. Svoboda, E.L.A., Shiga, A. and Deporter, D.A. (1981) A stereological analysis of collagen phagocytosis by fibroblasts in three soft connective tissues with differing rates of collagen turnover. *Anat. Rec.* 199, 473-480.

20. Melcher, A.H. and Chan, J. (1981) Phagocytosis and digestion of collagen by gingival fibroblasts *in vivo*: a study of serial sections. *J. Ultrastruc. Res.* 77, 1-36.

21. Keene, D.R., Sakai, L.W., Bachinger, H.P. and Burgeson, R.E. (1987) Type III collagen can be present in banded collagen fibrils regardless of fibril diameter. *J. Cell Biol.* 105, 2393-2402.

22. Bruns, R.R., Press, W., Engvall, E., Timpl, R. and Gross, J. (1986) Type VI collagen in extracellular, 100 nm periodic fibrils and filaments: identification by immunoelectron microscopy. *J. Cell Biol.* 103, 393-404.

23. Scott, J.E. and Orford, C.R. (1981) Dermatan sulphate-rich proteoglycan associates with rat tail tendon collagen in the d band in the gap region. *Biochem. J.* 197, 213-216.

24. Carson, D.D., Dutt, A. and Tang, J.P. (1987) Glycoconjugate synthesis during early pregnancy: hyaluronate synthesis and function. *Dev. Biol.* 120, 228-235.

25. Bell, S.C., Hales, M.W., Patel, S., Kirwan, P.H. and Drife, J.O. (1985) Protein synthesis and secretion by the human endometrium and decidua during early pregnancy. *Br. J. Obstet. Gynaecol.* 92, 793-803.

26. Bulmer, J.N. and Johnson, P.M. (1984) Macrophage populations in the human placenta and amniochorion. *Clin. Exp. Immunol.* 57, 393-403.

27. Campbell, E.J., Cury, J.D., Lazarus, C.J. and Welgus, H.G. (1987) Monocyte procollagenase and tissue inhibitor of metalloproteinases. *J. Biol. Chem.* 262, 15862-15868.

28. Jones, P.A. and Scott-Burden, T. (1979) Activated macrophages digest the extracellular matrix produced by cultured cells. *Biochem. Biophys. Res. Commun.* 86, 71-77.

29. Parakkal, P. (1969) Involvement of macrophages in collagen resorption. *J. Cell Biol.* 41, 345-354.

30. Gross, J. (1981) An essay on biological degradation of collagen. In: "Cell Biology of Extracellular Matrix". Editor: E.D. Hay, Plenum, New York, pp 217-258.

31. Zorn, T.M.T., Bevilacqua, E.M.A.F. and Abrahamsohn, P.A. (1986) Collagen remodelling during decidualisation in the mouse. *Cell Tissue Res.* 244, 443-448.

32. Van Veen, H.A. and Peereboom-Stegeman, J.H.J.C. (1987) The influence of the estrous cycle on the volume density and appearance of collagen-containing vacuoles in fibroblasts of the rat uterus. *Virchows Arch. B.* 57, 23-31.

33. Ruoslahti, E. (1988) Fibronectin and its receptors. *Annu. Rev. Biochem.* 57, 375-413.

34. Zardi, L., Carnemolla, B., Siri, A., Petersen, T.E., Paolella, G., Sebastio, G. and Baralle, F.E. (1987) Transformed cells produce a new fibronectin isoform by preferential alternative splicing of a previously unobserved exon. *EMBO J.* 6, 2337-2342.

35. Vartio, T., Laitinen, L., Narvanen, O., Cutolo, M., Thornell, L-E., Zardi, L. and Virtanen, I. (1987) Differential expression of the ED sequence-containing form of cellular fibronectin in embryonic and adult human tissues. *J. Cell Sci.* 88, 419-430.

36. Wewer, U.M., Faber, M., Liotta, L.A. and Albrechtsen, R. (1985) Immunochemical and ultrastructural assessment of the nature of the

pericellular basement membrane of human decidual cells. *Lab. Invest.* 53, 624-633.

37. Faber, K., Wewer, U.M., Berthelson, J.G., Liotta, L.A. and Albrechtsen, R. (1986) Laminin production by human endometrial stromal cells relates to the cyclic and pathological state of the endometrium. *Am. J. Pathol.* 124, 384-391.

38. Roberts, R., Gallagher, J., Spooncer, E., Allen, T.D., Bloomfield, F. and Dexter, T.M. (1988) Heparin sulphate bound growth factors: a mechanism for stromal cell mediated haemopoiesis. *Nature* 332, 376-378.

39. Pollard, J.W., Bartocci, A., Arceci, R., Orlofsky, A., Ladner, M.B. and Stanley, E.R. (1987) Apparent role of the macrophage growth factor, CSF-1 in placental development. *Nature* 330, 484-486.

40. Li, T.C., Roger, A.W., Lenton, E.A., Dockery, P. and Cooke, I.D. (1989) A comparison between two methods of chronological dating of human endometrial biopsies during the luteal phase, and their correlation with histological dating. *Fertil. Steril.* In press.

PARACRINE AND AUTOCRINE FACTORS INVOLVED IN THE REGULATION OF THE RELEASE OF HUMAN DECIDUAL PROLACTIN AND HUMAN PLACENTAL LACTOGEN

S. Handwerger, A. Golander, R. Richards, K. Thrailkill, V. Jorgensen, I. Harman and A. Grundis

Duke University, Durham, NC, USA

During pregnancy, the decidua and placenta synthesise and secrete several protein hormones that have identical or nearly identical chemical and biological properties to protein hormones synthesised and secreted by the pituitary gland and other tissues. For example, human decidual tissue synthesises and releases protein hormones that are identical to pituitary prolactin[1] and ovarian relaxin.[2] The placenta synthesises and releases hCG and hPL which have striking chemical and biological similarities to LH and to growth hormone and prolactin, respectively.[3] Nevertheless, despite the striking similarities between these hormones, the regulation of the synthesis and secretion of the protein hormones from the decidua and placenta is different from that of the pituitary protein hormones. Pituitary prolactin, growth hormone and most protein hormones are stored in large secretory granules, but ultrastructural and biochemical studies indicate that decidual prolactin[4] and hPL[5] are localised in the post-microsomal supernatants of decidual and placental tissue homogenates.

We report here studies from our laboratory on the regulation of the synthesis and release of decidual prolactin and placental prolactin and present new evidence indicating novel regulatory pathways involved in the release of these hormones. Particular attention will be given to the role of autocrine and paracrine factors in the regulation of decidual prolactin.

DECIDUAL PROLACTIN

Our initial studies of the synthesis and release of decidual prolactin indicated that TRH, dopamine, and bromocriptine had no effect on the synthesis or release of decidual prolactin, even at concentrations 1000 times the half-maximal concentrations that affect the synthesis and release of pituitary prolactin.[6] In addition, oestrogen[7] and vasoactive intestinal polypeptide (unpublished observation), both of which stimulate pituitary prolactin release, had no effect on the release of decidual prolactin.

Several studies subsequently demonstrated that exposure of endometrial tissue from the follicular phase of the menstrual cycle to progesterone resulted in decidualisation of the endometrium and in a striking increase in both the synthesis and release of prolactin.[8] Several investigators also observed that progesterone stimulated prolactin release from decidualised endometrium.[9] However, we were unable to demonstrate an effect of progesterone on prolactin synthesis or release from either decidual explants or monolayer cultures of decidual cells.[7]

Since our initial experiments clearly demonstrated that the regulation of the synthesis and release of decidual prolactin is different from that of pituitary prolactin, we next examined whether the release of decidual prolactin is affected by a factor or factors released by the placenta.[10] In our experiments we observed that decidual explants co-cultured for up to 24 hours with placental explants released more prolactin than decidual explants alone, and the magnitude of stimulation increased in proportion to the amount of placental tissue (Fig. 1). Exposure of decidual explants or cells to either human placental extracts or medium conditioned by human placenta (PCM) also resulted in a dose-dependent increase in prolactin synthesis and release. The stimulation by placental extracts and PCM was relatively specific for decidual prolactin, since neither placental extracts or PCM stimulated the release of total TCA-precipitable decidual proteins or the release of pituitary prolactin, LH, parathyroid hormone, and hPL. Moreover, conditioned medium from other human tissues, including skin fibroblasts, had no effect on the synthesis or release of decidual prolactin.

Initial chemical studies of the stimulatory factor(s) in placental extracts and PCM indicated that the stimulatory activity was not affected by dialysis (10 kD molecular weight cut off) or extraction with lipid solvents, but was completely blocked by trypsin and other proteolytic enzymes.[10] In subsequent investigations, we succeeded in purifying to homogeneity a single 23.5 kD protein in placental extracts and PCM that stimulates decidual prolactin release.[11] The purification scheme consisted

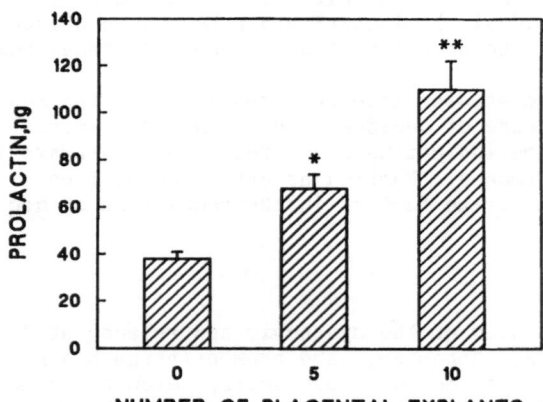

Figure 1.   The effects of placental tissue on the release of decidual prolactin. After a 24 h preincubation, decidual explants were incubated for 2 h in either control medium or medium containing either 5 or 10 placental explants. Each column represents the mean of triplicate cultures and the bars indicate + SEM. P vs control: *, p < 0.05; **, p < 0.01. Placental tissue incubated alone for 2 h released no detectable PRL. From Handwerger et al.[10]

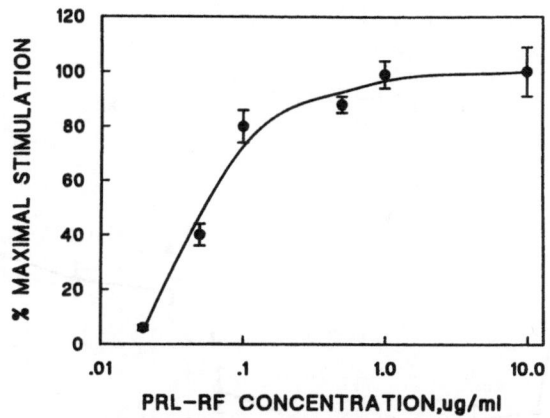

Figure 2. The dose-dependent effects of purified PRL-RF on prolactin release from human decidual explants. PRL-RF
that had been purified from PCM by DEAE-cellulose,
Spherogel TSK-3000, and immunoaffinity chromatographies
was assayed for prolactin releasing activity over 0.5
hour. Each point represents the mean of triplicate
cultures, and the bars show SEM. From Handwerger et
al.[11]

of ammonium sulphate fractionation, anion exchange chromatography, molecular sieve chromatography and immmunoaffinity chromatography with a polyclonal antiserum to the releasing factor. The purified releasing factor,
which we have designated decidual prolactin-releasing factor (PRL-RF),
stimulated the acute release of decidual prolactin within 30 minutes of
exposure with a half-maximal dose of 0.05 to 0.1 ug/ml (2.2 - 4.4 nM) as
shown in Figure 2.

Subsequent investigations demonstrated that, in addition to stimulating
an acute release of prolactin, PRL-RF also has a secondary and prolonged
effect on prolactin release beginning six to eight hours after exposure to
the releasing factor (Fig. 3). The acute stimulation by PRL-RF was
prevented by somatostatin but was unaffected by cycloheximide. On the other
hand, the secondary and delayed effect of PRL-RF was not blocked by
somatostatin but was completely prevented by cycloheximide, suggesting that
the delayed effect of PRL-RF was secondary to an increase in prolactin
synthesis.

More recent studies from our laboratory indicate that the synthesis
and release of decidual prolactin are also stimulated by IGF-I
(somatomedin-C) as shown in Figure 4. In these experiments, exposure of
decidual cells to IGF-I resulted in a dose-dependent stimulation of
prolactin synthesis and release (half-maximal concentration of 25 ng/ml)
beginning 48 - 72 hours after exposure. The binding of IGF-I to decidual
cells was blocked by α-IR₃, a monoclonal antibody to the IGF-I receptor,
and it completely inhibited the stimulation of prolactin release by IGF-I.
Conditioned medium of decidual cells contained only a very small concentration of IGF-I, suggesting that the decidua does not release IGF-I. Since
human placental tissue has been shown to synthesise and release IGF-I, it
is possible that placental IGF-I may be involved in the regulation of the
synthesis and release of decidual prolactin *in vivo*. Recent studies
indicate that decidual tissue releases a somatomedin binding protein, but
the effect of this binding protein on prolactin release is unknown.

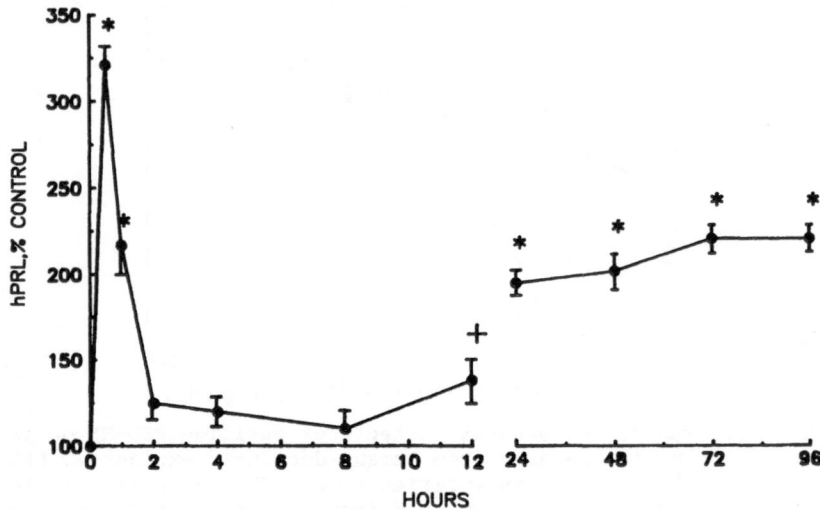

Figure 3. The acute and secondary effects of PRL-RF on decidual prolactin release. After a 48 h preincubation in control medium, decidual cells were exposed to PRL-RF (0.5 ug/ml) or control medium for 96 h with medium changes at the end of each 24 h interval. Aliquots (100 ul) were removed from the media at 0.5, 1, 2, 4, 8, and 12 h and replaced with an equal volume of medium of the same composition. The amounts of PRL released by the PRL-RF-exposed cells at each time are expressed as a percentage of the PRL released by control cells. Each point represents the mean + SEM of four cultures. P vs control: +, P < 0.05; *, P < 0.01. From Golander et al.[12]

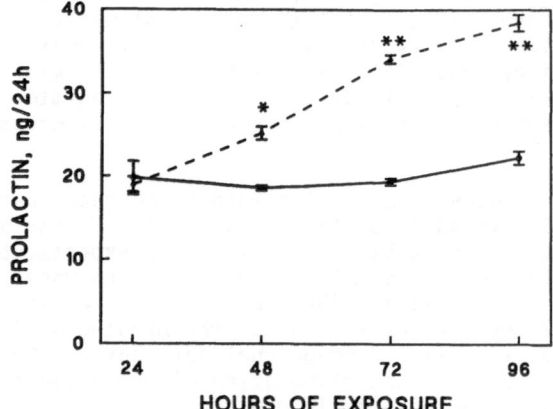

Figure 4. The effect of IGF-I on decidual prolactin release. After a 48 h preincubation in control medium, decidual cells were exposed for 96 h to control medium (o —— o) or medium containing IGF-I at a concentration of 200 ng/ml (▲ ---- ▲). Each point represents the mean + SEM of triplicate cultures. P vs control: *, P < 0.05; **, P < 0.01.

Studies by Huang and co-workers[13] have demonstrated that relaxin, a protein hormone with striking similarities to IGF-I and insulin, stimulates the release of prolactin from human endometrial stromal cells. Stromal cells exposed to relaxin released two to three times as much prolactin as control cells, and the stimulation was enhanced by progesterone and oestrogen. Since immunofluorescent studies strongly suggest that relaxin and prolactin are synthesised and released by the same decidual cells, the demonstration that relaxin stimulates decidual prolactin release is another example of autocrine control of hormone release.

Numerous studies from our laboratory indicate that the regulation of the synthesis and release of decidual prolactin is under negative as well as positive (PRL-RF, IGF-I) control. While exposure of decidua to placental conditioned medium stimulates decidual prolactin release, exposure of decidual cells or explants to conditioned medium from human decidual tissues results in a specific dose-dependent inhibition of prolactin release (Fig. 5).[14] The inhibition of prolactin release, however, is not due to negative feedback by prolactin, since removal of the prolactin in decidual conditioned medium by immunoprecipitation did not prevent the inhibitory effect. Furthermore, chromatographic analysis of decidual conditioned medium on Sephadex G-150 indicated that the inhibitory factor(s) has an apparent molecular weight of 45 kD while prolactin has a molecular weight of 23.5 kD. Partially purified preparations of the inhibitory factor, which we have designated as decidual prolactin-inhibitory factor (PRL-IF), not only inhibit the basal release of prolactin but also inhibit the stimulatory effects of PRL-RF on prolactin release.

At present the intracellular mechanisms involved in the regulation of the synthesis and release of decidual prolactin are unknown. However, several studies from our laboratory indicate that a number of second messengers may be involved in the regulation of the synthesis and release of prolactin. A role for cyclic AMP as a second messenger is strongly suggested by experiments demonstrating that exposure of decidual explants or cells to dibutyryl cyclic AMP, to the phosphodiesterase inhibitors IBMX, and theophylline, or to the adenylate cyclase activators cholera toxin and

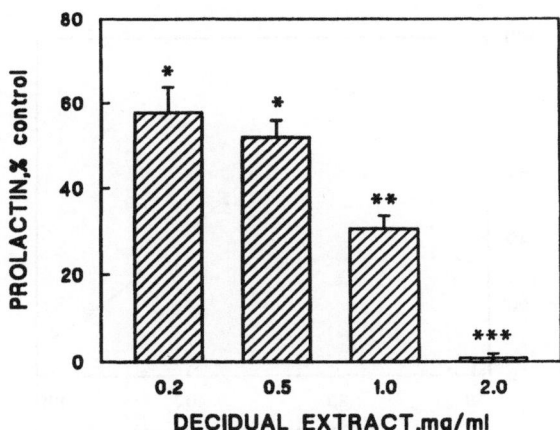

Figure 5. The effects of decidual extract on the release of decidual PRL. Triplicate cultures of decidual explants were incubated for 0.5 h in medium containing various concentrations of a decidual extract. Each point represents the mean + SEM of triplicate cultures. P vs control: *, P < 0.05; **, P 0.01; ***, P 0.005. From Markoff et al.[14]

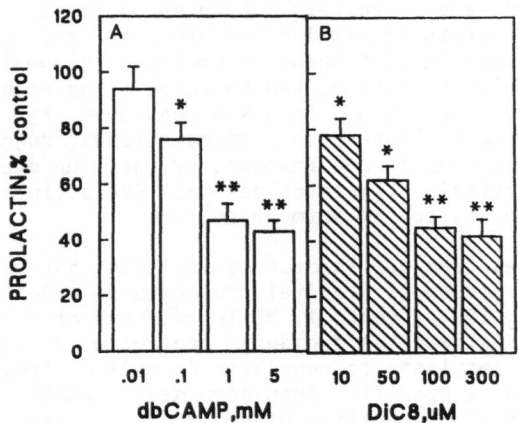

Figure 6.   The effects of dibutyryl cAMP (A) and sn-1,2-dioctanoyl-
            glycerol (diC8) (B) on decidual prolactin release. After
            2 h of incubation in serum-free medium, decidual cells
            were exposed for 0.5 h to either control medium or
            medium containing dibutyryl cAMP or dioctanoylglycerol.
            Results are expressed as % prolactin release relative to
            control cells.   Each bar represents the mean of tripli-
            cate cultures, and each bracket encloses 1 SEM. P vs
            controls: *, P < 0.05; **, P < 0.01. From [15], [16]

forskolin   cause dose-dependent inhibition of the synthesis and release of
prolactin (Fig. 6A).[15]   Subsequent   studies also suggest that activation of
phosphoinisotide hydrolysis may also be involved in the regulation of the
synthesis   and   release of prolactin (Fig.   6B).[16] Activation   of   protein
kinase C by either synthetic diacylglycerols or by phorbol esters resulted
in a significant dose-dependent inhibition of the synthesis and release of
prolactin.   On the other hand, phorbol esters and acylglycerols that do not
stimulate protein kinase C were without effect.

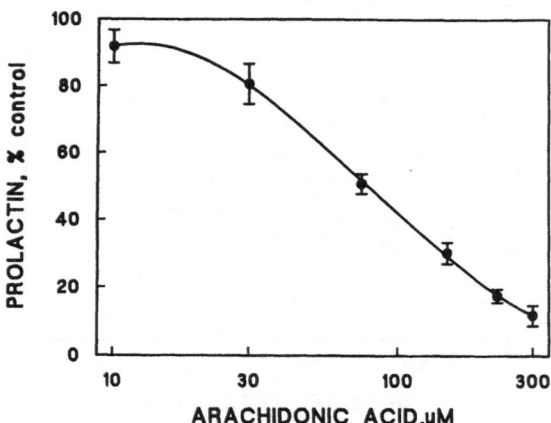

Figure 7.   The dose-dependent effect of arachidonic acid on pro-
            lactin release from human decidual explants. After a 24
            h incubation in serum-free medium, decidual explants
            were   exposed for 0.5 h to arachidonic acid   at
            concentrations from 0 - 300 um. The results are the
            mean of triplicate cultures.   The brackets enclose 1
            SEM. From Handwerger et al![8]

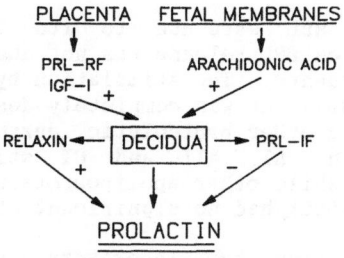

PLACENTA   FETAL MEMBRANES

PRL-RF   ARACHIDONIC ACID
IGF-I +   +

RELAXIN ◄─── DECIDUA ──► PRL-IF
         +   ─

PROLACTIN

Figure 8.   A schematic representation of the regulation of prolactin release from human decidua.

Arachidonic acid may also be a second messenger in the synthesis and
release of decidual prolactin (Fig. 7).[16] Exposure of decidual explants or
cells to arachidonic acid results in a specific, rapid, and reversible
dose-dependent inhibition of the synthesis and release of prolactin. The
inhibition, however, is not prevented by either cyclo-oxygenase or lipo-
oxygenase inhibitors, which seems to indicate that the inhibition may be
due to arachidonic acid itself or to some, as yet, unidentified arachidonic
acid metabolite. Since almost all of the intracellular arachidonic acid is
derived from the cleavage of arachidonic acid from the sn-2 position of
plasma membrane phospholipids by phospholipase A_2, it is possible that some
of the factors which regulate decidual prolactin may do so by modulating
phospholipase A_2 levels. Plasma arachidonic acid concentrations increase
during pregnancy, so it is also possible that arachidonic acid may act as a
first messenger in the synthesis and release of decidual prolactin.

A proposed model for the regulation of the synthesis and release of
decidual prolactin is summarised in Figure 8. The synthesis and release of
decidual prolactin are stimulated by PRL-RF, a 23.5 kD protein released by
the placenta, and by IGF-I, which is released by the placenta and other
tissues. PRL-RF has both an acute and a delayed effect on the synthesis and
release of prolactin with the delayed effect evident by six to eight hours
after exposure. The stimulation of prolactin release by IGF-I, on the other
hand, is not evident until 48 - 72 hours after exposure. The synthesis and
release of decidual prolactin is inhibited by PRL-IF, a 45 kD protein
released by the decidua, and arachidonic acid which is released by the
fetal membranes.[17] Several second messengers may be involved in prolactin
release: cyclic AMP, inositol trisphosphate, diacylglycerol, and arachidonic acid.

PLACENTAL LACTOGEN

Although hPL has striking chemical and biological similarities to
growth hormone and prolactin, the synthesis and release of hPL does not
appear to be regulated by such factors as insulin-induced hypoglycaemia,
hyperglycaemia, growth hormone-releasing factor, somatostatin, dopamine or
bromocriptine.[3] Recent studies from our laboratory strongly suggest that
the synthesis and release of hPL may be regulated, at least in part, by
several novel factors including high density lipoproteins (HDL)[18] and an
hPL-releasing protein found in serum from pregnant women.[19]

Initially we examined the effects of HDL on hPL release because of the
observations that placental plasma membranes contain specific HDL receptors[20] and HDL and hPL concentration in plasma increase concomitantly
during pregnancy.[21] We found that exposure of placental explants or cells
to HDL resulted in a dose-dependent stimulation of hPL release with half-
maximal stimulation occurring at 250 mg/ml which is within the normal
physiological range (Fig. 9). Although previous studies indicated that the

biological functions of HDL were due to its lipid constituents the biological action of HDL on PRL release was not due to lipids but due to the apolipoprotein constituents. The stimulation by HDL was not decreased by lipid extraction of HDL, but was completely destroyed by proteolytic digestion with trypsin and other proteolytic enzymes. In addition, the delipidated apolipoproteins AI, AII and CI stimulated dose-dependent increases in PRL release while other apolipoproteins were without effect. Low density lipoproteins (LDL) had no significant effect on PRL release.

More recent studies from our laboratory indicate that HDL also stimulates PRL secretion *in vivo*.[22] Administration of sheep HDL to pregnant ewes at 80 - 140 days of gestation at a dose of 102 - 700 mg caused a dose-dependent stimulation of PRL secretion, while administration of much larger amounts of non-HDL plasma proteins were without effect. Since HDL and hPL concentrations increase concomitantly during pregnancy and trophoblast cells contain HDL receptors, the *in vivo* and *in vitro* effects of HDL on hPL release is strong evidence for a physiological role of HDL in the regulation of PRL release during pregnancy.

In recent studies, we have found that several synthetic peptide analogues of the amphipathic helical structure of the apolipoproteins also stimulate hPL release. The magnitude of the stimulation of hPL release in response to the analogue peptides correlated with the ability to displace apolipoproteins from HDL and with other measures of phospholipid binding affinity such as the increase in helicity and the size of complexes formed between the peptide and phospholipid. The correlation of stimulatory ability and lipid affinity suggests that the action of the apolipoproteins on hPL release may be mediated through an interaction with plasma membrane phospholipids.

Earlier investigations from our laboratory indicated that pharmacological agents which increase intracellular cAMP levels also stimulate hPL release.[23] To examine whether cAMP might be a second messenger in HDL-mediated hPL release, we investigated whether HDL stimulates cAMP levels in human trophoblast cells and adenylate cyclase in placental membranes.[24]

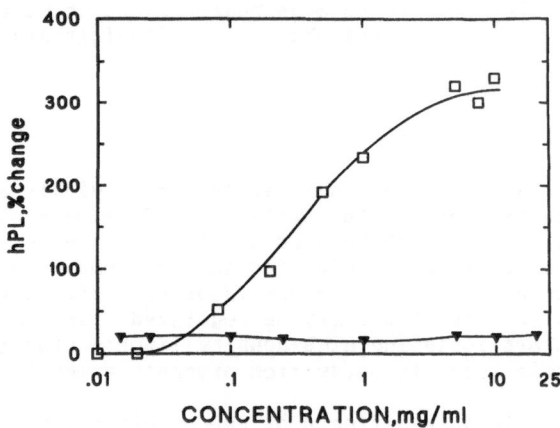

Figure 9.   The effects of high and low density lipoproteins on hPL
release. Human placental cells were exposed for 1 h to
HDL (open squares) or LDL (closed triangles). Each
point represents the mean of triplicate cultures. From
Barrett et al.[19]

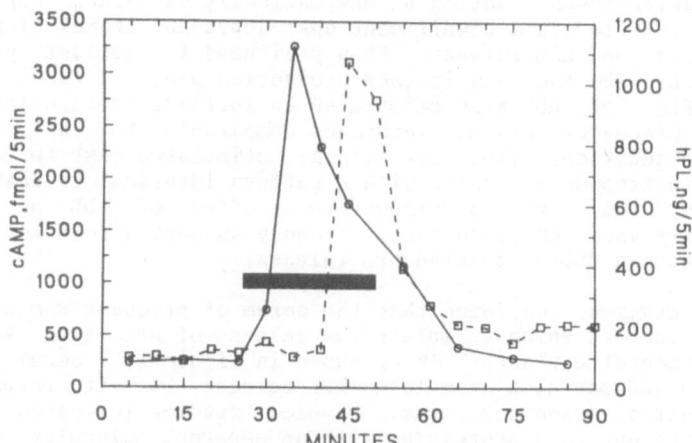

Figure 10. The effects of HDL on the release of cAMP and hPL from perifused human trophoblast cells. After 25 min perifusion with control medium, trophoblast cells (6 x 10 cells/chamber) were exposed to HDL (150 ug/ml) for 25 min (solid bar). At the end of the period of time, cells were again perifused with control medium. The results of cAMP (o —— o) and hPL (□ ---- □) are expressed as fmol/5 min and ng/5 min, respectively. The flow rate during the entire perifusion period was 6 ml/h and the medium was collected in 5 min/fraction. From Wu et al[24]

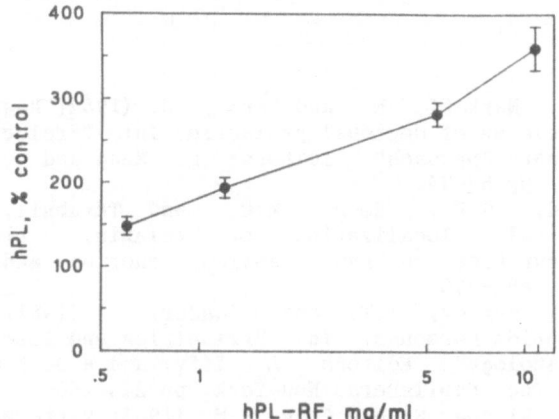

Figure 11. The dose-dependent effect of human pregnancy serum on hPL release from perifused trophoblast cells. After a 2 h preincubation, perifused trophoblast cells (5 x 10/chamber) were exposed for 6 h to control medium or medium containing a pool of human pregnancy serum at concentrations of 0.6, 1.2, 5.4, or 10.8 mg/ml. Modified from.[25]

Exposure of an enriched fraction of enzymatically dispersed hPL-producing cells to HDL resulted in a significant dose-dependent stimulation of both cAMP production and hPL release. When perifused trophoblast cells were exposed to HDL, the increase in cAMP production preceded the increase in hPL release (Fig. 10). HDL also stimulated an increase in adenylate cyclase activity in placental plasma membranes comparable to that caused by adrenalin. In addition, apolipoprotein AII stimulated cAMP formation and hPL release in trophoblast cells with a pattern identical to that of HDL. These results, the first to demonstrate an effect of HDL on adenylate cyclase activity and cAMP production, strongly suggest a role for cAMP as a second messenger in HDL-stimulated hPL release.

In other studies, we found that the serum of pregnant women contains one or more factors which stimulate the release of hPL from trophoblast cells and placental explants[19,20] as shown in Figure 11. Serum from non-pregnant women and men also stimulated hPL release, but with potencies only about 10% that of pregnancy serum. Chemical studies indicated that the stimulation was due to a protein(s) with an apparent molecular weight of approximately 35 kD. At present, the site of synthesis of the hPL-releasing factor is unknown.

In summary, studies from our laboratory lead us to believe that the synthesis and release of prolactin from human decidual cells is regulated, at least in part, by factors released by the placenta and fetal membranes and by paracrine or autocrine factors. The synthesis and release of hPL appears to be regulated, at least in part, by HDL, apolipoproteins AI, AII, and CI, and a releasing factor that is present in the serum of pregnant women.

Acknowledgements

We thank Janet Barrett, Susan Barry, Edith Markoff, Philip Zeitler, Yun Qi Wu, Mae Harris, Linda Pierce, and Larry Kodack for their many contributions to these studies. We thank Gayle Kerr for secretarial assistance. Supported by NIH grants HD15201 and HD07447.

REFERENCES

1. Handwerger, S., Markoff, E. and Barry, S. (1984) Regulation of the synthesis and release of decidual prolactin. In: "Prolactin Secretion: A Multidisciplinary Approach". Editors: F. Mena and C.M. Valverde, Academic Press, pp 57-74.
2. Bryant-Greenwood, G.D., Rees, M.C. and Turnbull, A.C. (1987) Immunohistochemical localization of relaxin, prolactin and prostaglandin synthase in human amnion, chorion and decidua. J. Endocrinol. 114, 491-496.
3. Handwerger, S., Hurley, T.W. and Golander, A. (1981) Placental and decidual polypeptide hormones. In: "Principles and Practice of Obstetrics and Perinatology". Editors: L. Iffy, and H.D. Kaminetzky, John Wiley and Sons, Inc. Publishers, New York, pp 243-260.
4. Handwerger, S., Wilson, S. and Conn, P.M. (1984) Different subcellular storage sites for decidual- and pituitary-derived prolactin: possible explanation for differences in regulation. Mol. Cell. Endocrinol. 37, 83-87.
5. Handwerger, S., Wilson, S.P., Tyrey, L. and Conn, P.M. (1987) Biochemical evidence that human placental lactogen and human chorionic gonadotropin are not stored in cytoplasmic secretion granules. Biol. Reprod. 37, 28-32.
6. Golander, A., Barrett, J., Hurley, T., Barry, S. and Handwerger, S. (1979) Failure of bromocriptine, dopamine and thyrotropin-releasing

hormone to affect prolactin secretion by decidual tissue *in vitro. J. Clin. Endocrinol. Metab.* **49,** 787-789.

7. Markoff, E., Zeitler, P., Peleg, S. and Handwerger, S. (1983) Characterization of the synthesis and release of prolactin by an enriched fraction of human decidual cells. *J. Clin. Endocrinol. Metab.* **56,** 962-968.

8. Daly, D.C., Maslar, I.A. and Riddick, D.H. (1982) Prolactin production during *in vitro* decidualization of proliferative endometrium. *Am. J. Obstet. Gynecol.* **145,** 672-678.

9. Daly, D.C., Maslar, I.A. and Riddick, D.H. (1983) Term decidua response to estradiol and progesterone. *Am. J. Obstet. Gynecol.* **145,** 679-683.

10. Handwerger, S., Barry, S., Markoff, E., Barrett, J. and Conn, P.M. (1983) Stimulation of the synthesis and release of decidual prolactin by a placental polypeptide. *Endocrinology* **112,** 1370-1374.

11. Handwerger, S., Capel, D., Korner, G. and Richards, R. (1987) Purification of decidual prolactin-releasing factor, a placental protein that stimulates prolactin release from human decidual tissue. *Biochem. Biophys. Res. Commun.* **147,** 452-459.

12. Golander, A., Richards, R., Thrailkill, K., Capel, D., Rogers, D. and Handwerger, S. (1989) Decidual prolactin-releasing factor stimulates the synthesis of prolactin from human decidual cells. *Endocrinology* In press.

13. Hung, J.R., Tseng, L., Bischoff, P. and Janne, O.A. (1987) Regulation of prolactin production by progestin, estrogen, and relaxin in human endometrial stromal cells. *Endocrinology* **121,** 2011-2017.

14. Markoff, E., Howell S. and Handwerger, S. (1983) Inhibition of decidual prolactin release by a decidual peptide. *J. Clin. Endocrinol. Metab.* **57,** 1282-1286.

15. Handwerger, S., Harman, I., Costello, A. and Markoff, E. (1987) Cyclic AMP inhibits the synthesis and release of prolactin from human decidual cells. *Mol. Cell. Endocrinol.* **50,** 99-106.

16. Harman, I., Costello, A., Ganong, B., Bell, R.M. and Handwerger, S. (1986) Activation of protein kinase C inhibits synthesis and release of decidual prolactin. *Am. J. Physiol.* **251,** E172-E177.

17. Handwerger, S., Barry, S., Barrett, J., Markoff, E., Zeitler, P., Cwikel, B. and Siegel, M. (1981) Inhibition of the synthesis and secretion of decidual prolactin by arachidonic acid. *Endocrinology* **109,** 2016-2021.

18. Handwerger, S., Quarfordt, S., Barrett, J. and Harman I. (1987) Apolipoproteins AI, AII, and CI stimulate placental lactogen release from human placental tissue. A novel action of high density lipoprotein apolipoproteins. *J. Clin. Invest.* **79,** 625-628.

19. Barrett, J., Golander, A., Conn, P.M. and Handwerger, S. (1986) Characterization and partial purification of a serum protein which stimulates the release of human placental lactogen *in vitro. J. Clin. Endocrinol. Metab.* **63,** 336-342.

20. Winkel, C.A., Gilmore, J., MacDonald, P.C. and Simpson, E.R. (1980) Uptake and degradation of lipoproteins by human trophoblastic cells in primary culture. *Endocrinology* **107,** 1892-1898.

21. Desoye, G., Schweditsch, M.O., Pfeiffer, K.P., Zechner, R. and Kostner, G.M. (1987) Correlation of hormones with lipid and lipoprotein levels during normal pregnancy and postpartum. *J. Clin. Endocrinol. Metab.* **64,** 704-712.

22. Grandis, A., Jorgensen, V., Kodack, L. and Handwerger, S. (1989) High density lipoproteins (HDL) stimulate placental lactogen secretion in pregnant ewes: Further evidence for a role of HDL in placental lactogen secretion during pregnancy. *J. Endocrinol.* In press.

23. Harman, I., Costello, A., Sane, A. and Handwerger, S. (1987) Cyclic adenosine-3',5'-monophosphate stimulates the acute release of placental lactogen from human trophoblast cells. *Endocrinology* **121,** 59-63.

24. Wu, Y.Q., Jorgensen, E.V. and Handwerger, S. (1989) High density lipoproteins stimulate placental lactogen release and adenosine 3':5'-

cyclic monophosphate production in human trophoblast cells: Evidence for cyclic AMP as a second messenger in hPL release. *Endocrinology* In press.

25. Sane, A., Harman, I., Costello, A., Quarfordt, S. and Handwerger, S. (1988) Characterization of placental lactogen release from perifused human trophoblast cells. *Placenta* 9, 129-138.

PLACENTA AS A SOURCE

EDITORIAL INTRODUCTION

There is no organ that can be compared with the placenta when we consider it as a source. Whether delivered as an abortus or at full term, we hold in our hands a mass of diverse tissue from which we can derive inter alia, nucleic acids, lectins, growth factors and hormones.

Lectins would appear to be ubiquitous in nature, so their presence in early as well as in full term placenta comes as no surprise. Their relevance and role - for example, in the initiation of specific cellular responses or release of immunoregulatory substances - is still matter for investigation and discussion, as Margita Čuperlović and Miroslava Janković explain in their paper.

Growth factors are presently much in the limelight. Tissue-specific growth factors which are questionably different are isolated from the most varied sources at regular intervals, and reported with almost equal regularity in the learned journals. What is their importance? Are they all species and tissue specific? These questions and others are addressed in the paper by Hugo Burgos, and in that of Olga Genbačev and her colleagues. In both we learn at once there is nothing new in the realisation that the placenta and its membranes possess "healing properties", and Burgos describes how these properties of amniotic membrane may be defined and utilised.

Genbačev and her colleagues go a stage further by making an extract of early trophoblast and testing its action on experimentally-inflicted eye lesions in rabbits and chronic ulcers in man. Angiogenesis, as a result of injection or application of the cytosol extract, can be seen by the naked eye; granulation and epithelialisation follow hard on its heels. Such observations make a case for the presence of these factors (or possibly a single, all-embracing, factor) in the early placenta. Isolation, purification, characterisation, and synthesis are the next problems to be solved in the investigation of these putative factors. But these are technical matters, which undoubtedly patience, time and skill will eventually overcome.

For the reader it may be a major step simply to appreciate that the placenta, like the fetus which arises from the same cell as itself, is a microcosm of all man's vital processes.

ENDOGENOUS β-GALACTOSIDE BINDING LECTIN OF HUMAN PLACENTA

Margita Čuperlović and Miroslava Janković

Institute of Endocrinology, Immunology and Nutrition
INEP, Zemun, Yugoslavia

An ever-increasing interest in lectins - carbohydrate-binding proteins of nonimmune origin that agglutinate cells or precipitate glycoconjugates[1] - has resulted in the discovery and isolation of many lectins from plants, bacteria, non-vertebrate and vertebrate tissues, and body fluids. The accumulation of data on lectin existence in nearly all classes of living organisms so far examined seems to imply that they may represent an ancient evolutionary system, still well adapted to the performance of specific functions - presumably through the recognition and binding of glycoconjugates.

The capacity of lectins to precipitate glycoconjugates, agglutinate cells, and stimulate lymphocyte blastogenesis *in vitro* has been used in many laboratories for more than 20 years. However, their physiological functions have been recognised only recently, and are not yet completely understood.

VERTEBRATE LECTINS

Initial evidence that vertebrate tissues and body fluids contained saccharide-binding proteins emerged from the examination of fish agglutinins.[2] Soon after, the existence of a β-D-galactoside binding protein with lectin properties was demonstrated in a variety of mammalian tissues.[3] The search for lectin activities in various animal and human tissues resulted in the isolation and characterisation of many, more or less related, lectins. This led to the prediction in 1982[4] that lectins may be present in all cells, although their activities may vary greatly on account of development, specific cell function, and tissue differentiation, for example.

The recognised vertebrate lectins are divided roughly into two classes: integral membrane lectins, which require detergents for extraction from the tissue, and readily extractable soluble lectins.[5] This tentative classification is not purely technical, but implies certain differences of function. Membrane-bound lectins may be involved in the attachment of glycoproteins to plasma membrane or in their intracellular translocation - or both, while soluble lectins are secreted from cells and interact with soluble extracellular or insoluble membrane-bound glycoconjugates.

The existence of this class of sugar-binding proteins was invoked to explain the role of glycoprotein carbohydrate moieties before the lectins were identified and isolated. The best example is a hepatic asialoglyco-protein receptor.[6] The first intimation of the existence of such a lectin came from accumulated experimental data indicating that desialysation of serum glycoproteins accelerated their hepatic clearance.[7] Liver plasma membranes were found to be the major loci of binding for desialylated serum proteins with exposed galactose or N-acetylgalactosamine residues. Subse-quently, the receptor was isolated and purified from Triton X-100 extracts of rabbit, rat, and human livers by affinity chromatography on asialo-orosomucoid Sepharose.[8-10] The receptor was characterised and designated as a lectin, based on the criteria that it would induce erythrocyte agglutination and lymphocyte mitosis *in vitro*. It was established that the asialoglycoprotein receptor is a transmembrane glycoprotein which mediates the binding and internalisation of glycoproteins with terminal galactose or N-acetylgalactosamine residues. The process of receptor-mediated endocyto-sis involves binding of circulating asialoglycoproteins and internalisation of the receptor-ligand complex into the cell, where the ligand is degraded and the receptor recycled back to the plasma membrane.[11,12] The activity of asialoglycoprotein is maximal in mature, nonproliferating differentiating hepatocytes and decreases in developing, regenerating preneoplastic and neoplastic liver as a result of a post transcriptional mechanism.[13]

Other membrane-bound lectins have also been isolated from mammalian livers, such as the surface receptor of Kupffer cells, specific for mannose/N-acetylglucosamine;[14] fucose-binding protein;[15] and phosphoman-nosyl receptor predominantly located intracellularly.[16]

Recognition systems for glycoconjugates, governed by membrane-bound lectins, are not the exclusive property of the liver. Similar or immunologically identical lectins have been isolated from other tissues. However, the expression of their activity varies greatly not only in terms of localisation, but also at different developmental stages of the same tissue.[17-19] The first experimental data indicating that human placental tissue also contains membrane-bound lectins with various specificities appeared recently. Using histochemical methods Gabius et al[20] identified several sugar-binding proteins in human placenta. Some of these were isolated by affinity chromatography on columns with immobilised carbohy-drates, but have not yet been completely examined and characterised. They are mostly detergent soluble, Ca^{2+} dependent and α-fucoside specific, and localised in the trophoblast layer of the placenta. The physiological significance of these membrane-bound lectins and where they fit in the complex metabolic processes of the human placenta remain to be explained.

SOLUBLE VERTEBRATE LECTINS

The other group of vertebrate lectins, tentatively classified according to their solubility, comprises the ubiquitous family of closely related proteins found in aqueous extracts of various tissues and cells. The first to be isolated and purified were lectins from the electric organ of the electric eel[3] and from the calf heart and lung,[21] while the most extensively studied were two β-galactose-binding lectins found in the intestine and other tissues of embryonic and adult chickens.[22,23] Subse-quent developments in this field have been rapid.[5,24,25] Soluble lectins have been isolated from muscle, regenerating liver, brain, retina and other tissues of embryonic chickens, from mice tissues, and from tissues of amphibia and reptiles. Human tissues also contain soluble lectins of this type. They have been found in human muscle,[26,27] lung,[28] spleen,[29] placenta,[30] and in tumour cells of various origin.[31,32]

Most soluble lectins presently known belong to a closely related family of β-galactoside-specific proteins. The basic properties characteristic of this group, also termed galaptines, are: - haemagglutinating activity that can be inhibited by β-galactoside-containing compounds; structural similarity expressed by the presence of subunits with M_r falling between 12 and 16 k Daltons that often contain identical epitopes; the requirement of a sulphydryl reagent, but not metal ions, for full activation; possible developmental regulation of activity; readily solubilisation in the absence of detergent by buffers containing lactose.

Soluble lectins with such characteristics have been localised both extra- and intra-cellularly. Shift of lectin localisation from being predominantly intracellular to extracellular is connected with embryonic development and post-natal maturation of tissues.[33] Consequently, an extracellular role of lectins has been suggested.[25]

HUMAN PLACENTAL LECTIN - HP-14

Taking into account the general features of soluble lectins, it seems likely that they will be involved in the metabolic processes of the placenta. Most of the pregnancy-associated and pregnancy-specific proteins are glycoproteins with a strongly expressed sugar component.[34] Urinary excretion of oligosaccharides increases in pregnancy,[35] indicating that a saccharide tag is more pronounced in placental synthetic products. Additionally, some of the developmentally regulated soluble trophoblast products have properties which are attributes of lectins, such as the ability to bind to polysaccharides[34] or induce immunodeviations.[36] Extracts of pregnancy urine and crude commerical hCG preparations contain a contaminant that is mitogenic for human peripheral blood lymphocytes and behaves differently from purified hCG or growth factors.[37] In addition, pregnancy itself is followed by a redistribution of glycoconjugates exposed on the surface of specific cells. Damjanov and Lee have shown by means of plant lectin histochemistry that glycosilated cell surface constituents of the placenta, endometrium, and other pregnancy-related tissues appear or disappear in an ordered and stage-specific manner.[38,39] This provides the basis for suggesting that during embryonic development, as well as during malignant transformation, the presence and developmental changes of sugar receptors may lead to specific carbohydrate-protein (lectin) interactions. These could have a physiological significance in connection with the organisation of cells and their response to regulatory factors.

Isolation and Composition of Human Placental Lectin

The first unequivocal identification of a soluble placental lectin was made by Hirabayashi and Kasai, who described the structure, properties and some biological and immunological activities of the lectin in which they had isolated.[30,33] Human placental lectin was isolated from extracts of trophoblast, using the same method originally developed for isolating chicken intestinal lectin.[22]

The method consists of homogenisation of placenta in 20 mM sodium phosphate buffer, pH 7.2, containing 150 mM NaCl, 4 mM 2-mercaptoethanol and 2 mM EDTA (EDTA-MEPBS). The lectin is isolated from the undissolved portion by EDTA-MEPBS, supplemented with 0.1 M lactose which releases lectin from the glycoconjugate to which it was bound originally. After removal of the lactose by gel filtration or dialysis, lectin is isolated by affinity chromatography on a column of asialofetuin-Sepharose 4B. Lactose (20 mM) in EDTA-MEPBS buffer is used again for desorption (Figure 1).

This preparation seemed homogeneous on SDS-polyacrylamide gel electrophoresis. However isoelectric focusing produced multiple bands around pH

147

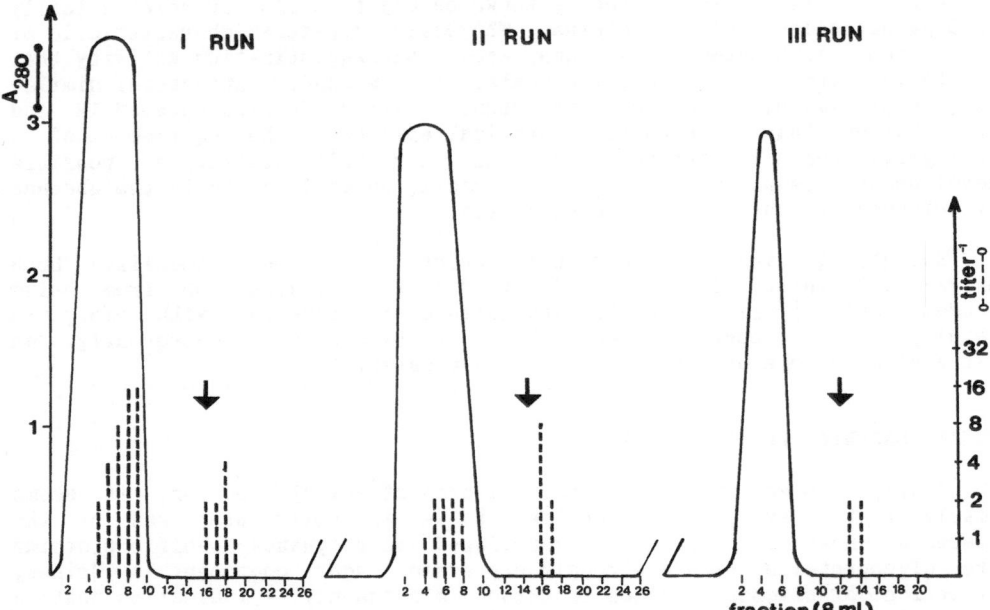

Figure 1.   Human placental lectin (HP-14) separation on asialofetuin-Sepharose 4B column (1.2 x 11 cm).   Extracts of
placental proteins were run repeatedly through the
affinity column. Elution was performed with EDTA-MEPBS
buffer, with the addition of 20 mM lactose from
fractions marked (arrow).   Haemagglutinating activity
was determined with trypsin-treated rabbit erythrocytes
and expressed as titre.

5, with a major band at pH 4.9.[34] Oligometric structure, as determined by
high-performance gel filtration, corresponded to monomer (14 kD) and dimer
(28 kD), and both forms were present in the lectin preparations.

Human placental lectin, designated HP-14, possesses a low haemagglutinating activity for trypsinised rabbit erythrocytes.   Saccharide-binding
specificity has been examined in the usual way by measuring the inhibitory
effect of various saccharides on the lectin-haemagglutinating activity.
The highest affinity is for thiodigalactoside and lactose.   No metal
requirement for full lectin activity has been found.

The amino acid composition of HP-14 (Table I) is characterised by a low
cysteine content.   This was underestimated at first and then found to be 5
free SH-residues per subunit.[34] The haemagglutinating activity of HP-14 is
lost in the absence of 2-mercaptoethanol, as thiol groups are evidently
involved in the saccharide-binding sites of this and other β-galactoside
binding lectins.

The overall amino acid composition of HP-14 is similar in composition
to some of the other vertebrate lectins already mentioned.   In addition,
determination of the primary structure of HP-14[23] showed it has a blocked
N-terminal and some regions that are highly homologous to the corresponding
segments of chick 14 K lectin.   Genes that encode human dimeric β-
galactoside-binding lectin containing M_r = 14 subunits, like the subunit of
HP-14, have been isolated.[36]   It was suggested they comprise a family of at

Table I. Amino acid composition of β-galactoside binding lectin of human placenta (HP-14)[30]

Amino Acid	Molar Ratio
Aspartic Acid	22.6
Threonine	1.7
Serine	5.8
Glutamic Acid	10.5
Proline	5.5
Glycine	12.4
Alanine	13.1
Cysteine*	0.94
Valine	9.3
Methionine	0.96
Isoleucine	3.8
Leucine	11.5
Tyrosine	1.7
Phenylalanine	8.8
Lysine	7.4
Histidine	1.9
Arginine	4.8
Tryptophane	0.4

* Cysteine corrected to five free residues per subunit[34]

least three genes, which would explain the structural diversity of β-galactoside-binding lectins isolated from various human tissues and the microheterogeneity of HP-14. The investigation of the immunological crossreactivity between HP-14 and other β-galactoside binding lectins confirmed a relationship between HP-14, mouse 15 K, chick 14 K and chick 16 K lectins.

On the basis of the relationships between the known β-galactoside-binding proteins, a hypothesis was proposed that four epitopes are characteristic of these vertebrate lectins.[23] Each lectin contains two out of four possible epitopes, which are characteristic of mammalian (A), chick (B), monomer-type (C), and dimer-type (D) lectins. The distribution of the characteristic epitopes in some of the lectins mentioned, including HP-14, would be as shown in Table II. Each characteristic epitope is connected with some functional property of the lectin - for example, haemagglutinating activity, or the degree of thiol dependence. Lectins containing the same epitopes are immunologically cross-reactive. According to this hypothesis, HP-14 would be classified as mammalian monomer-type β-galactoside-binding protein with a weak haemagglutinating activity.

Although HP-14 has now been purified and characterised, very little is known of its biological properties and function in the placenta. It has been found in first trimester and full term placenta, although there are differences in its activity and concentration.

Placental proteins insoluble in EDTA-MEPBS, but solubilised after the addition of lactose, possess, as explained earlier, a haemagglutinating activity characteristic of HP-14. This haemagglutinating activity of the extracted proteins has been used as a rough indicator of the lectin activity in the trophoblast (Table III). The concentration of proteins extracted with EDTA-MEPBS lactose from early placenta was less than that of

Table II. Distribution of characteristic epitopes among the related vertebrate β-galactoside binding lectins[23]

Lectin	Characteristic Epitope	
Human HP-14	A	C
Chick 14 K	B	C
Chick 16 K	B	D
Mouse 15 K	A	D

Table III. Haemagglutinating activity of the EDTA-MEPBS lactose extracts of the placenta

	First Trimester Placenta	Term Placenta
No. of samples	15	8
Concentration of extracted proteins (mg/ml)	0.45 ± 0.11	1.87 ± 0.42
Haemagglutinating activity:		
HU/mg wet tissue	0.08 ± 0.025	0.12 ± 0.04
HU/mg protein	36 ± 7.8	12.7 ± 3

HU is defined as the lowest protein concentration that provides clear haemagglutination of trypsine-treated rabbit erythrocytes.

All values are expressed as the Mean ± SD.

proteins extracted from the same amount of term placenta. Haemagglutinating activities of proteins originating from first trimester placenta were, however, about three times higher, indicating that extracts of early placenta contain more lectin compared with other proteins that might be present, or that this lectin was in a more active form.

Recently it has been found that β-galactoside-specific lectin of rat lung can be present in a more or less active form, and that activation of the lectin and its turnover can be modulated hormonally.[37] This provides some interesting opportunities for speculation on the possibility and significance of hormonal regulation of lectin activity during gestation.

Role of Placental Lectin

A possible function for HP-14 in processes taking place in the placenta itself or governed by products of the placenta during gestation remains to

be determined. Lectin activity found in crude preparations of hCG obtained
from the urine of pregnant women or in the blood obtained from umbilical
cord indicates that lectin synthesised in the trophoblast circulates
freely, not only in the placenta, but also in the maternal circulation and
possibly in fetal fluids.   Based on the data obtained for other β-
galactoside specific soluble lectins, there may be three main directions of
activity. These are tissue organisation, the organisation of complex
glycoconjugates, and immunological functions.

During pregnancy saccharide-containing cell surface components of
pregnancy-related tissues increases dramatically, as shown by lectin
histochemistry,[38,39] thus indicating that lectins may be involved in cell-
cell adhesion and tissue organisation.   So far, similar activity has been
established for CLL-I and erythroid developmental agglutinin.[25] There is
also the possibility that HP-14 may, like CLL-II and several other soluble
lectins, be involved in the extracellular organisation of mucous secretory
products.

More precise immunohistochemical localisation of HP-14 and identification of specific glycoconjugates with which it associates in the trophoblast would help draw a distinction between these two possible directions
of HP-14 involvement in extracellular organisation.

Another possible biological function of HP-14 in connection with its
immunomodulatory effects has been investigated. Placenta is known to
contain several immunoregulatory proteins that are immunosuppressive or
immunostimulant, and produce an immunodeviatory situation characteristic of
pregnancy.[36]   There are experimental data indicating that HP-14 could be
included among the immunomodulatory proteins.   In vitro HP-14 can induce
release of a cytotoxin from a murine macrophage cell line and human
monocytes alike.[33] Other soluble vertebrate lectins are involved, again in
vitro, in the lectin-dependent cytotoxicity of lymphocytes and macrophages.
These show a broad target affinity characteristic of lectins.   It has been
suggested that lectin-mediated cytotoxicity may occur in vivo through
mediation by lectins that may be present in body fluids.[39]   Immunosuppressive effects of lectins have also been detected, expressed by
generation of potent suppressor cells capable of inhibiting activities of T
and B cells in vitro, or retarding graft rejection in vivo. Lectins are
thought to be capable of promoting negative, as well as positive,
modulations of lymphocyte activity, because these activities are exercised
through particular areas on the surface of the cell, and triggered by the
binding of lectin.[39]

It may be summarised fairly confidently that human trophoblast contains
a soluble β-galactoside specific lectin, characterised by weak haemagglutinating activity for trypsin-treated rabbit erythrocytes, which does not
require metal ions for its full activity, and occurs as a monomer (M_r = 14
kD) or dimer. This has been detected in early and full term placentae with
some concentration differences in relation to other proteins extracted
under similar conditions.   The biological functions of this protein could
be related to its ability to bind β-galactoside-containing glycoconjugates
exposed on the cell surface or present extracellularly, leading to cell-
cell adhesion and tissue organisation, the aggregation of soluble glycoconjugates or the initiation of specific cellular responses, such as the
release of immunomodulatory substances.

The precise direction of HP-14 activity and many aspects of its
relationships with other active proteins of the placenta remain to be
investigated.   The results should contribute to a better understanding of
the complex processes governed by the placenta and the still unclear
biological functions of soluble β-galactoside-binding proteins in general.

REFERENCES

1. Goldstein, I.J., Hughes, R.C., Monsigny, M., Osawa, T. and Sharon, N. (1980) What should be called a lectin? *Nature* **285**, 66.
2. Lis, H. and Sharon, N. (1972) Lectins: cell-agglutinating and sugar-specific proteins. *Science* **177**, 949-959.
3. Teichberg, V.I., Silman, I., Beitsch, D.D. and Resheff, G. (1975) A beta D-galactoside binding protein from electric organ tissue of Electrophorus electricus. *Proc. Natl. Acad. Sci. USA.* **72**, 1383-1387.
4. Olden, K., Parent, J.B. and White, S.L. (1982) Carbohydrate moieties of glycoproteins. A re-evaluation of their function. *Biochim. Biophys. Acta.* **650**, 209-232.
5. Barondes, S.H. (1984) Soluble lectins: a new class of extra-cellular proteins. *Science* **223**, 1259-1264.
6. Pricer, W.E. and Ashwell, G. (1971) The binding of desialylated glycoproteins by plasma membranes of rat liver. *J. Biol. Chem.* **246**, 4825-4833.
7. Morrell, A.G., Gregoriadis, G., Scheinberg, I.H., Hickman, J. and Ashwell, G. (1971) The role of sialic acid in determining the survival of glycoproteins in the circulation. *J. Biol. Chem.* **246**, 1461-1467.
8. Kawasaki, T. and Ashwell, G. (1976) Chemical and physical properties of an hepatic membrane protein that specifically binds asialoglycoprotein. *J. Biol. Chem.* **251**, 1296-1302.
9. Tanabe, T., Pricer, W.E. and Ashwell, G. (1979) Subcellular membrane topology and turnover of a rat hepatic binding protein specific for asialoglycoprotein. *J. Biol. Chem.* **254**, 1038-1043.
10. Baeziger, J.A. and Maynard, Y. (1980) Human hepatic lectin. *J. Biol. Chem.* **255**, 4607-4613.
11. Ashwell, G. and Harford, J. (1982) Carbohydrate-specific receptor of the liver. *Annu. Rev. Biochem.* **51**, 531-554.
12. McFarlane, I.G. (1983) Hepatic clearance of serum glycoproteins. *Clin. Sci.* **64**, 127-135.
13. Hubert, B.E., Glowinski, I.B. and Thorgirsson, S.S. (1986) Transcriptional and post-transcriptional regulation of the asialoglycoprotein receptor in normal and neoplastic rat liver. *J. Biol. Chem.* **26**, 12400-12407.
14. Maury, C.P. (1983) Hepatic lectins. Concept, biochemistry and role. *Scand. J. Gastroenterol.* **18**, 321-325.
15. Gabius, H.J., Debbage, P.L., Engelhardt, R., Osmer, S.R. and Lange, W. (1987) Identification of endogenous sugar-binding proteins (lectins) in human placenta by histochemical localization and biochemical characterization. *Europ. J. Cell Biol.* **44**, 265-272.
16. De Waard, A., Hickman, S. and Kornfeld, S. (1976) Isolation and properties of beta galactoside-binding lectins of calf heart and lung. *J. Biol. Chem.* **251**, 7581-7587.
17. Beyer, E.C., Zweig, S.E. and Barondes, S.H. (1980) Two lactose binding lectins from chicken tissues. *J. Biol. Chem.* **255**, 4236-4239.
18. Beyer, E.C. and Barondes, S.H. (1982) Secretion of endogenous lectin by chicken intestinal goblet cells. *J. Cell Biol.* **92**, 28-33.
19. Barondes, S.H. (1981) Lectins: their multiple endogenous cellular functions. *Annu. Rev. Biochem.* **50**, 207-231.
20. Barondes, S.H. (1986) The Lectins. Properties, Functions and Applications in Biology and Medicine. Editors: I.E. Liever, N. Sharon, and I.J. Goldstein, Academic Press. pp 457-466.
21. Powell, J.T. (1980) Purification and properties of lung lectin. *Biochem. J.* **187**, 123-129
22. Allan, H.J., Cywinski, M., Palmberg, R. and Di Ciocco, R.A. (1987) Comparative analysis of galactose-binding lectins isolated from mammalian spleens. *Arch. Biochem. Biophys.* **250**, 523-533.
23. Hirabayashi, J., Oda, Y., Oohara, T., Yamagata, T. and Kasai, K. (1989) Immunological cross-reactivity between beta glactoside-binding

lectins of vertebrates. Possible relationship of antigenicity to oligomeric structure. *Biochem. Biophys. Acta*. In press.

24. Gabius, H-J., Engelhardt, R., Rehm, S. and Cramer, F. (1984) Biochemical characterization of endogenous carbohydrate binding proteins from spontaneous murine rhamdomyosarcoma, mammary adenocarcinoma and ovarian teratoma. *J. Natl. Cancer Inst*. **73**, 1349–1357.

25. Gabius, H-J., Engelhardt, R., Casper, J., Schmoll, J., Nagel, G.A. and Cramer, F. (1985) Comparison of endogenous lectins in human embryonic carcinoma and yolk sac carcinoma. *Tumour Biol*. **6**, 471–482.

26. Joubert, R., Caron, M. and Bladier, D. (1987) Brain lectin-mediated agglutinability of dissociated cells embryonic and postnatal mouse brain. *Brain Res*. **36**, 146–150.

27. Bohn, H. (1985) Biochemistry of placental proteins. In: "Proteins of the Placenta". Editors: P. Bischof and A. Klopper, Karger, Basel, pp 1–25.

28. Derappe, C., Bauvy, C. and Lemonnier, M. (1986) Isolation and characterization of two sialyloligosaccharides containing N-acetyl-lactosamine from pregnancy urine. *Carbohyd. Res*. **145**, 341–347.

29. Voisin, G.A., Duc, H.T. and Bobe, P. (1985) Immunomodulatory proteins of the placenta. In: "Proteins of the Placenta". Editors: P. Bischof and A. Klopper, Karger, Basel, pp 54–67.

30. Morse, J.H., Ehrlich, P.H. and Canfield, R.E. (1982) Extracts of pregnancy urine contain a mitogen for human peripheral blood lymphocytes (PBL). *J. Immunol*. **128**, 2187–2193.

31. Damjanov, I. and Lee, I. (1986) Pregnancy-related changes in murine and human endometrium revealed by differential binding of fluorescei-nated lectins in pregnancy. In: "Pregnancy Proteins in Animals". Editor: J. Hau, Walter de Gruyter, Berlin, pp 177–183.

32. Lee, M.C. and Damjanov, I. (1984) Lectin histochemistry of human placenta. *Differentiation* **28**, 123–128.

33. Kajikawa, T., Nakajima, Y., Hirabayashi, J., Kasai, K. and Yamazaki, M. (1986) Release of cytotoxin by macrophages on treatment with human placenta lectin. *Life Sci*. **39**, 1177–1181.

34. Hirabayashi, J., Kawasaki, H. Suzuki, K. and Kasai, K.I. (1987) Further characterization and structural studies on human placenta lectin. *J. Biochem*. **101**, 987–995.

35. Hirabayashi, J. and Kasai, K. (1984) Human placenta beta galactoside binding lectin. Purification and some properties. *Biochem. Biophys. Res. Commun*. **122**, 938–944.

36. Gitt, M.A. and Barondes, S.H. (1986) Evidence that a human soluble beta galactoside-binding lectin is encoded by a family of genes. *Proc. Natl. Acad. Sci. USA*. **83**, 7603–7607.

37. Clerch, L.B., Whitney, P.L. and Massaro, D. (1987) Rat lung lectin synthesis, degradation and activation. *Biochem. J*. **245**, 683–690.

38. Bychkov, V. and Toto, P.D. (1986) Lectin binding to normal human endometrium. *Gynecol. Obstet. Invest*. **22**, 29–33.

39. Lis, H. and Sharon, N. (1986) The Lectins. Properties, Functions and Applications in Biology and Medicine. Editors: I.E. Liever, N. Sharon and I.J. Goldstein, Academic Press, pp 266–285.

THE PURIFICATION AND CLINICAL APPLICATION OF ANGIOGENIC AND GROWTH FACTORS

FROM HUMAN PLACENTA AND ENDOMETRIUM: POSSIBLE AUTOCRINE-PARACRINE ROLE

H. Burgos

Blond McIndoe Centre for Medical Research
East Grinstead, Sussex

Extra-embryonic membranes have been used from time to time in the treatment of burns, ulcers, and denuded areas in general with varying degrees of success and, sometimes, negative and contradictory results.[1-6] Amniotic epithelium from human amniochorion membrane maintained in culture[7] has been used in the treatment of chronic ulceration of the legs with remarkable success.[8,9] The application of this amniotic epithelium stimulated production of vascular granulation tissue within three to five days. These clinical observations were confirmed by histological examination. Biopsies taken before application of amnion epithelium presented, in general, a picture of dense connective tissue with thick reticulin fibres isolating few groups of thick walled capillaries having ill-defined endothelium. After amnion application, an increased number of thin-walled capillaries with well delimited endothelium were uniformly distributed between delicate connective tissue fibres. No amniotic epithelium was seen, as this is lysed in the ulcer bed 24 - 28 hours after application.[10] No rejection episode was ever observed, which confirms the lack of HLA expression in amnion.

High molecular weight components from Sephacryl S-300 gel filtration, previously called placental growth factors (PGFs), have been incorporated into dressings for topical application in the treatment of chronic varicose ulcers.[10] Geliperm (Geistlich, Wolhunsen, Switzerland), an agar polyacrylamide membrane dressing, and K-Y jelly (Johnson & Johnson Ltd., UK), a hydroxyethyl cellulose were used. The PGF-Geliperm dressings were applied to large ulcers, for which hospital admission and skin grafting were required. PGF-KY jelly was used in the treatment of small ulcers, not larger than 30 cm² area. These patients were not hospitalised. These applications produced a marked increase in granulation and epithelial tissue, and a significant percentage ulcer size reduction (37.2%), including complete healing, in small ulcers.

These clinical and histological results suggest there is a release of biologically active components from the amnion membrane. To investigate their nature and origin the following procedures were undertaken: placentae and amniochorion membranes were collected from elective Caesarean sections at term and the different anatomical entities were separated by blunt dissection and individually maintained in a serum and additive-free culture system.[7] Conditioned media were collected, and presence of biological activities demonstrated.[11] Angiogenic activity was demonstrated by chorioallantoic membrane (CAM) and subcutaneous implant (SCI) assays. Mitogenic activity was estimated by ^{3}H-thymidine uptake in cultures of normal, unstimulated peripheral blood lymphocytes and serum-starved 3T3 fibroblasts.

All the anatomical entities – chorion, adherent decidua, reflected and placental amnion, and trophoblast - showed biological activity.[11] Figure 1 illustrates the biological activity of placenta-conditioned media on 3T3 fibroblast cultures. Selective ultrafiltration through membranes of different molecular weight cutoff showed the presence of a variety of molecular size components (5 - 100 kD) exhibiting biological activities.

Gel filtration chromatography of amniochorion-conditioned medium was carried out in Sephacryl S-300.[11] The highest biological activity was in the first eluted peaks, detected at 280 nm, and corresponding to an area of the chromatogram where the molecular weight exceeded 100 kD. These high molecular weight components showed gradual loss of activity on dialysis in cellulose membranes (14 - 20 kD nominal molecular weight cutoff). The diffusates, however, exhibited biological activities. When high molecular weight components were submitted to high salt concentrations (2 M $MgCl_2$), then dialysed in small pore size membranes (2 kD cutoff), and the diffusates fractionated in a DE-52 cellulose chromatography column, the resultant components showed biological activity.[11] From these results it seems that high molecular weight components of conditioned medium are amenable to dissociation or disaggregation yielding intermediate size components with biological activities as well as active factors of less than 2 kD molecular weight.

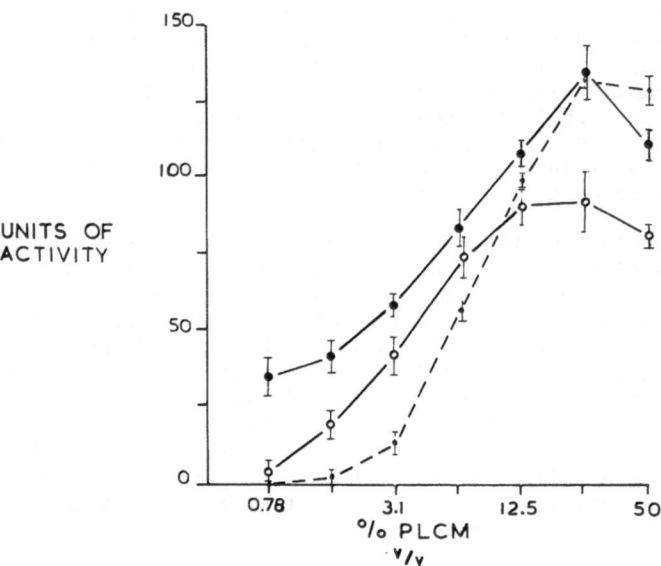

Figure 1.   Biological activity of term placenta conditioned media on serum starved 3T3 fibroblast cultures. Placenta conditioned media from 1st day (●——●) and 3rd day (o——o) cultures, and fetal calf serum (o - - - o). Each point represents the mean ± SEM of triplicate cultures, the ordinate, units of mitogenic activity and the abscisa, concentrations of conditioned media and fetal calf serum.

To purify and characterise the active factors, extracts of whole placentae, including amniochorion membranes and adherent decidua, have been prepared, and different components isolated by ion-exchange chromatography in DEAE-Sepharose CL6B. The highest biological activity corresponded with a small peak in the chromatogram, representing less than 1% of the protein content of the original sample, and eluting at the very beginning of the salt gradient. Fractionation of this peak by gel filtration chromatography in Sephacryl S-300 yielded two areas of activity well apart from each other in the chromatogram. A first area corresponded to "high molecular weight" components, eluting within the fractionation range of the gel and readily detected at 280 nm. A second area corresponded to "low molecular weight" components, retarded by hydrophobic interactions, eluting later and detected at 200 - 220 nm.[12] Low molecular weight components were isolated by reverse phase high performance liquid chromatography (HPLC) yielding a single, homogeneous peak, placental angiogenic factor (PAF). Amino acid analysis of this peak after 6 M HCl hydrolysis for 24 hours showed the presence of serine, glycine, alanine and lysine at a ratio 1:1:2:1. A molecular weight of 480 was found by fast atom bombardment mass spectrometry.[12] Amino acid sequencing studies have been unsuccessful so far because PAF presents a blocked N-terminus. A second peak, eluting later in the chromatogram, is present especially in scaled up preparations. This peptide, also biologically active, appears to be formed mainly of methionine, and presents a blocked N-terminus as well. Figure 2 shows separation of these peptides by reverse phase HPLC.

An angiogenesis factor of 18.7 kD that stimulates production of plasminogen activator and latent collagenase, DNA synthesis, and chemotaxis in cultured bovine capillary endothelial cells has also been purified from human term placenta by heparin-affinity chromatography.[13-15] This appears to be a polypeptide of the basic fibroblast growth factor class.[16]

Angiogenic factors have been isolated from first trimester human decidua by ultrafiltration through micropore membranes of 30 kD cutoff, followed by concentration on a 5 kD cutoff membrane.[17] In collaboration with Dr. E.S. Lindenbaum (Israel Institute of Technology, Haifa), these factors were used with dermis allograft carriers in surgically inflicted skin wounds in the rat. Preliminary results of these experiments showed increased neovascularisation and accelerated incorporation of the dermal grafts.

DISCUSSION

Experimental and clinical studies have demonstrated initiator, additive, and synergistic effects of trophoblast angiogenic and growth promoting factors.[10-12] Trophoblast and endometrium angiogenic factors appear to be useful tools for acceleration and modulation of wound healing. However, there is not yet enough information about the molecular structure of these factors, their site of synthesis and genomic expression, their target cell receptors, and their mechanisms of action, interaction, regulation and control. Circumstantial evidence suggests a possible involvement of placenta-endometrium angiogenic factors in autocrine-paracrine regulation.

Angiogenesis occurs normally during embryonic development, endometrial regeneration, and wound healing. A menstrual period is a kind of physiological wound and the implantation of an embryo could be regarded in the same light. Of course there are differences between the loss of endometrial tissue at menstruation and the destruction of the decidua involved in implantation. The rapid growth of the trophoblast results in continuous destruction and repair of decidual tissue. This in turn causes

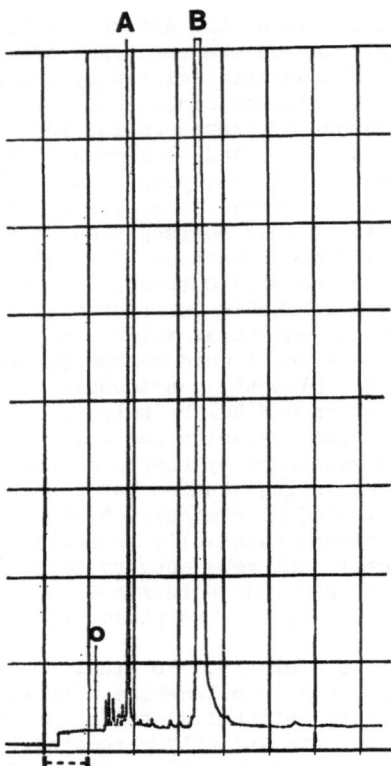

Figure 2.   Separation of low molecular weight placental angiogenic
peptides (A and B) by high pressure liquid chromatography on Spherisorb C8 (4.6 x 10 cm). Isocratic
elution was carried out with 25 mmol/l triethylammonium
phosphate pH 2.5 at a flow rate 0.5 ml/min. (0 denotes
0 minutes, |----| equals 1 minute).

remodelling and regeneration of capillaries and larger blood vessels, in a
manner analogous to wound healing. The angiogenic factors involved in wound
healing may also play a part in endometrial regeneration. Cellular
proliferation and the growth of the placenta and uterus, on the other hand,
could not depend exclusively on diffusion mechanisms. Experimental studies
have shown that diffusion of growth hormones has an extremely short range
of penetration,[18] and cell growth in the endometrial membrane of the uterus
in the pregnant rat is restricted to a narrow zone, no more than 30 μm away
from the nearest capillary vessel.[19] The need for an autocrine-paracrine
system of angiogenesis for placenta-uterine growth becomes apparent.
Furthermore, a continuous supply of angiogenic factors must be maintained
to prevent regression of angiogenesis. Regression of de novo formed
capillaries is a common observation in experimental assays when angiogenic
factors are removed or inactivated.[11] The localised effect and in situ
activity of placenta and endometrium angiogenic factors also suggest an
autocrine-paracrine role.

Other growth promoting factors, such as epidermal growth factor and
fibroblast growth factor - both found in human placenta[20,21] - may exhibit
angiogenic activities in placenta and endometrium under certain
circumstances. Many cell types have a multiplicity of receptors to respond
to the appropriate growth promoting factors required for co-ordinate

growth.[22] In addition, some degree of crossreactivity for receptor recognition and/or further processing may take place temporarily to cope with any disturbance in the supply of specific growth factors. Alternative pathways of angiogenesis must be available in some neovascular processes not involving autocrine-paracrine mechanisms.

Acknowledgement

This work was supported by grants from the East Grinstead Medical Research Trust and Johnson & Johnson Ltd.

REFERENCES

1. Davis, J.S. (1910) Skin transplantation with a review of 550 cases at the Hopkins Hospital. *Johns Hopkins Hosp. Rep.* **15**, 307-395.
2. Stern, W. (1913) The grafting of preserved amniotic membrane to burned and ulcerated skin surfaces substituting skin grafts. *JAMA* **13**, 973-974.
3. Robson, M.C. and Krizek, T.J. (1973) Amniotic membranes as a temporary wound dressing. *Surg. Gynecol. Obstet.* **136**, 904-906.
4. Notea, E., Hirschowitz, B., Karev, A. and Mahler, D. (1975) The use of lyophilised amnion to treat burns and skin defects. *Harefuah* **88**, 265-267.
5. Eldad, A., Stark, N., Anais, D., Golan, T. and Ben-Hur, N. (1977) Amniotic membranes as a biological dressing. *S.A. Mediese Tydskrif.* **51**, 272-275.
6. Gruss, J.S. and Jirsch, D.W. (1978) Human amniotic membrane: A versatile wound dressing. *Can. Med. Assoc. J.* **118**, 237-240.
7. Burgos, H. and Faulk, W.P. (1981) The maintenance of human amniotic membranes in culture. *Br. J. Obstet. Gynaecol.* **88**, 294-300.
8. Bennett, J.P., Matthews, R.N. and Faulk, W.P. (1980) The treatment of chronic ulceration of the legs with human amnion. *Lancet.* **i**, 1153-1156.
9. Faulk, W.P., Matthews, R.N., Stevens, P.J., Bennett, J.P. Burgos, H. and Hsi, B.L. (1980) Human amnion as an adjunct in wound healing. *Lancet* **i**, 1156-1158.
10. Burgos, H. (1987) Incorporation and release of placental growth factors in synthetic medical dressings. *Clin. Materials* **2**, 133-139.
11. Burgos, H. (1983) Angiogenic and growth promoting factors in human amniochorion and placenta. *Eur. J. Clin. Invest.* **13**, 289-296.
12. Burgos, H. (1986) Angiogenic factor from human term placenta. Purification and partial characterisation. *Eur. J. Clin. Invest.* **16**, 486-493.
13. Moscatelli, D.A., Presta, M., Mignetti, P., Ossowski, L., Mullins, D.E., Crowe, R.M. and Rifkin, D.B. (1985) Purification and biological activities of an angiogenic factor from human placenta. *Anticancer Res.* **5**, 618, (Abstract).
14. Moscatelli, D.A, Presta, M., Mignetti, P., Mullins, D.E., Crowe, R.M. and Rifkin, D.B. (1986) Purification and biological activities of an angiogenesis factor from human placenta. *Anticancer Res.* **6**, 861-863.
15. Moscatelli, D., Presta, M. and Rifkin, D.B. (1986) Purification of a factor from human placenta that stimulates capillary endothelial cell protease production, DNA synthesis, and migration. *Proc. Natl. Acad. Sci. USA.* **83**, 2091-2095.
16. Folkman, J. and Klagsbrun, M. (1987) Angiogenic factors. *Science* **235**, 442-447.
17. Lindenbaum, E.S., Beach, D. and Maroudas, N.G. (1988) Angiogenic activity of partially purified human uterine angiogenic factor (HUAF) (personal communication).
18. Maroudas, N.G. and Wray, S. (1984) Gradients in activation of nuclear chromation of growth during pregnancy. *Isr. J. Med. Sci.* **10**, 646.

19. Maroudas, N.G. (1985) Activation of nuclear chromation in stretch-dependent growth of tissues. *Connect. Tissue Res.* **13**, 217-225.
20. O'Keefe, E., Hollenberg, M.D. and Cuatrecasas, P. (1974) Epidermal growth factor. Characteristics of specific binding in membranes from liver, placenta, and other target tissues. *Arch. Biochem. Biophys.* **164**, 518-526.
21. Gospodarowicz, D., Cheng, J., Lui, G.M., Fujii, D.K., Baird, A. and Bohlen, P. (1985) Fibroblast growth factor in the human placenta. *Biochem. Biophys. Res. Commun.* **128**, 554-562.
22. Godfrey, D.G., George, W.D., Porteous, C., Neagle, G. and Pragnell, I. (1987) Epidermal growth factor in gynaecological tissue and fluid. *J. Cell. Biochem.* **5** (s11A), 26, (Abstract).

HUMAN TROPHOBLAST: A BIOLOGICAL AND CLINICAL DEMONSTRATION OF ITS WOUND HEALING AND TISSUE REPAIR PROPERTIES

Olga Genbačev,[1] Jasna Lesić,[2] Dragica Ljuština,[3] S. Mičić,[3] Nada Papić,[3] Mirjana Vučković,[1] and Rebecca Beaconsfield[4]

Zemun,[1] Zagreb,[2] Belgrade,[3] Yugoslavia; London,[4] England

Traditionally, the placenta with the fetal membranes and umbilical cord is treated as a mere by-product of the newborn baby. It seems little short of amazing that this harvest of human tissue delivered directly into the obstetricians' hands is usually promptly discarded by them. It is the largest biopsy of healthy human tissue we can ever hope to obtain - so why does it fail to arouse interest, and for what reason does it remain relatively unexplored? In our view, examining its possible value in clinical medicine is important, and in this chapter we investigate some of its therapeutic potential.

For many years it has been known that preparations of amniotic membrane are useful as wound dressings and to promote wound healing,[1-5] but the satisfactory results obtained still await a scientific explanation. We now know that placenta is a rich source of proteins having different biological activities, and evidence is accumulating that trophoblast cells produce growth factors and also contain their receptors.[6-15] However, little research has been carried out at the interface of basic science and clinical medicine in the field of tissue repair and wound healing. Investigation into the processes regulating cell growth and multiplication is progressing rapidly, and an ever-increasing body of evidence suggests that growth factors are involved in wound repair.[16] Much less progress has been made in producing appropriate models for study of the role of growth factors in wound healing in man. As there is no satisfactory animal model from which the stages of wound healing can be extrapolated to man investigators keep searching for a technique to serve in lieu. To exemplify the complexity of the problem it is sufficient to mention that some workers have proposed conducting systematic studies of wound healing in man by inducing wounds experimentally in the legs of normal volunteers.[17]

Placentas can be obtained at term or early from legal abortions. As the trophoblast from first trimester placentas is dissected free from decidual tissue much more easily than at term we have used early placenta to study the potential of its cytosol proteins in stimulating angiogenesis and epithelialisation in a classical animal model - the rabbit cornea.

CORNEAL WOUNDS IN RABBITS

The rabbit cornea is known to be an excellent model for studies of wound healing *in vivo*,[18,19] since the epithelial regrowth which occurs after trauma is easily observed. Additionally, its accessibility makes it an *in vivo* model of choice to study the process – and progress – of angiogenesis.[20] For this reason we chose it for our first investigation into the effects of placental extract on wound healing.

A preparation of cytosol extract from first trimester placenta was made as previously described,[21,22] and 0.5 mg of these cytosol proteins – freeze-dried and lyophilised – dissolved in 0.5 ml N saline used as a subconjunctival injection and as eye drops.

Thirty two rabbits had standard alkali lesions of the cornea produced in both eyes (Figs. 1 and 4). While making the injury, a piece of amnion was used to protect the rest of the eye. Treatment of the right eye started the next day with the subconjunctival injection of 0.5 mg of cytosol protein in 0.5 ml N saline. This was repeated daily for five days, after which the eye was irrigated four times a day with drops of the same solution for a further 10 days. The left (control) eye was treated with saline alone.

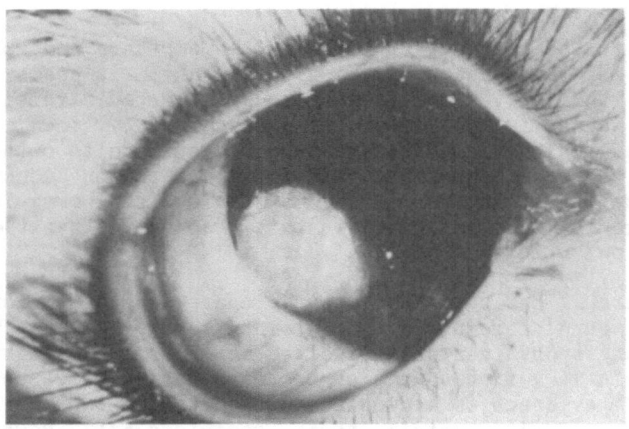

Figure 1.   Corneal lesion of right eye induced by alkali, 30 min after injury.

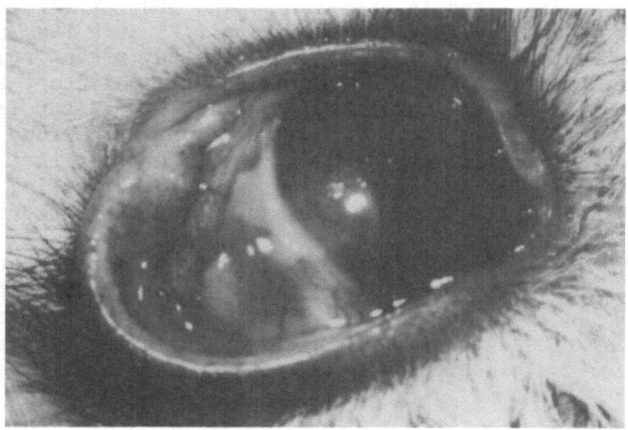

Figure 2.   Treated eye (right) 7th day after injury. Note decreased stromal opacity and newly formed capillary network at the site of injection.

Immediately after traumatisation the wounds appeared as white opaque patches in both eyes (Figs. 1 and 4). After seven days the opacity in the right (treated) eye had almost completely disappeared (Fig. 2). The opacity faded gradually in all treated eyes over a period of 15 days (Fig. 3). In the untreated group, in nine out of 12 rabbits only slight decrease in the opacity was observed at the periphery 15 days after injury, while the central area remained opaque (Fig. 5). The angiogenic effect of the extract is seen in Figure 6. Neovascularisation was maximal after nine days of treatment and appeared at the site of the injection. Small capillaries crossed the corneal limbal junction and penetrated the cornea. Twelve to 15 days after injury complete regression of these newly formed vessels was observed (Fig. 7).

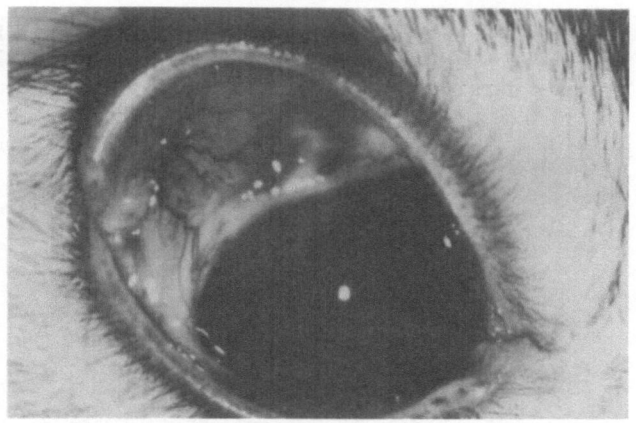

Figure 3.   Treated eye (right) 15 days after the injury. Complete disappearance of stromal opacity. Blood vessels seen at the site of injection.

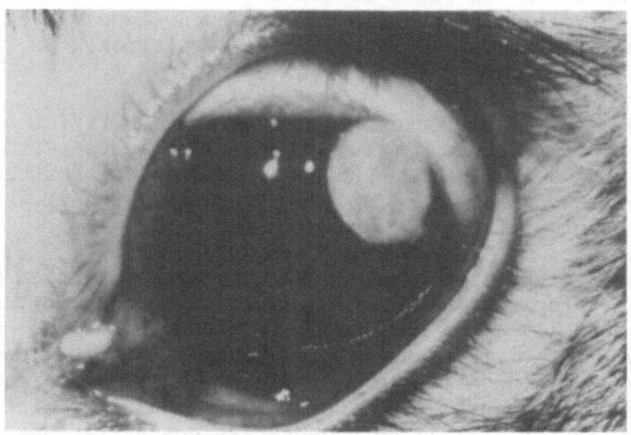

Figure 4.   Corneal lesion of left eye induced by alkali, 30 min after injury.

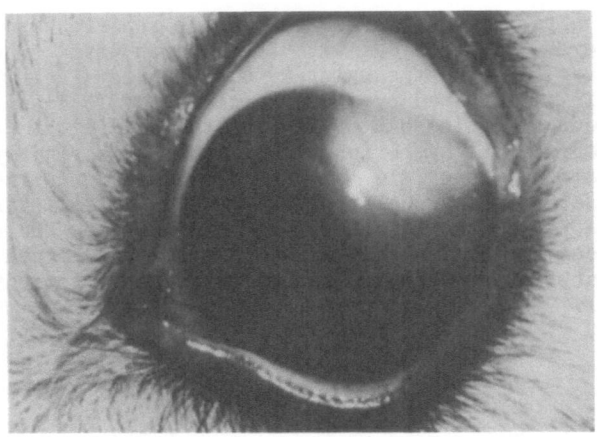

Figure 5.   Left eye (untreated) 15 days after the injury. Slightly decreased opacity at the periphery of wound;   elsewhere opacity persists.

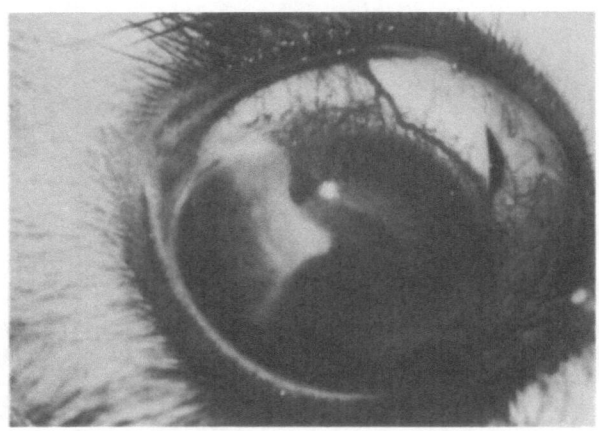

Figure 6.   Right eye; neovascularisation 9 days after injury.

Neovascularisation in wound repair is well documented as a transient stage of wound healing,[12] and the cornea would appear to follow this pattern. No side effects, such as local irritation, or any allergic reactions were observed.

The   success of this treatment encouraged us to try the effects of trophoblast cytosol fraction in two groups of patients with non-healing wounds of differing aetiology, but both well recognised for their intractability to treatment – namely, indolent (varicose) leg ulcers and post-irradiation chronic cystitis.

However, before starting treatment we introduced further precautionary measures into the preparation of the extract. Although a cytosol fraction by virtue of centrifugation is free of viral particles we screened our preparation for hepatitis B antigen and found it to be uncontaminated. Radioimmunoassays were negative for oestradiol and progesterone but showed the presence of the placental proteins hCG, hPL and SP_1 in the preparation. Albumen and thermostable alkaline phosphatase concentrations were too low to be detectable by routine clinical methods.

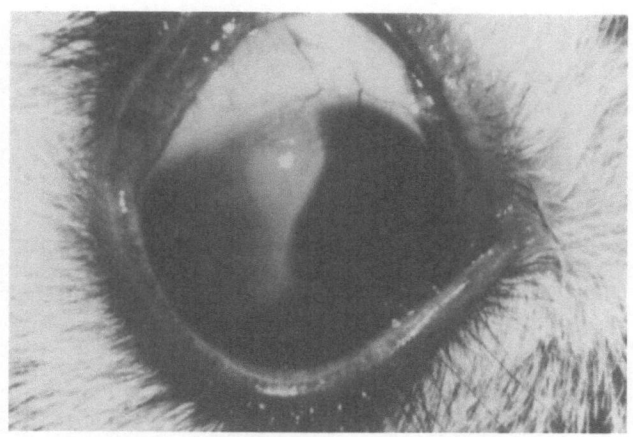

Figure 7. Regression of newly formed blood vessels at 12 days after injury.

INDOLENT LEG ULCERS

To treat the patients with leg ulcers the cytosol fraction was incorporated into an inactive vehicle, Lekobaza cream (Yugoslav Pharmacopoeia No. 053 180/4), in the proportion of 2 mg of cytosol proteins per 50 g of the cream.[22]

Our patients with leg ulcers consisted of a group of 165 persons, whose ages ranged from 37 to 76 years and who had been treated unsuccessfully by conventional methods for periods of from four months up to three years. The ulcers were varicose in origin, and all were in the region of the ankle. In some of these patients amputation was already being discussed as the only possible further treatment. In ten patients with bilateral ulcers informed consent was given to treat the second ulcer with Lekobaza cream alone. We were thus able to compare the effects of the vehicle with those of vehicle plus placental extract. These ten patients likewise had come to us after varying long periods of unsuccessful conventional treatment. None of the patients had any other disease, such as diabetes.

Before starting treatment each ulcer was measured and photographed (Fig. 8a is an example), and this procedure was repeated weekly. The patients remained hospitalised until their ulcers healed. At the first treatment the ulcer was gently debrided with normal saline, and the depth of the cavity noted; in many patients the cavity extended down to the bone. In cases where the slough was thick and adherent, and did not completely separate on the first occasion, debridement was repeated. The cleaned ulcer bed was then packed to the floor of the cavity with the extract-containing cream. This was repeated daily.

Blood samples were taken at weekly intervals and assayed for placental proteins (hPL, SP_1 and βhCG). Probably due to the poor vascularity of the ulcer bed, no placental proteins were found in these blood samples. There was no evidence of any systemic absorption from the cream, nor were there any systemic effects that could be attributed to its constituents.

Three time intervals were recorded for each patient, taking the start of treatment as day 1. The time intervals were: day 1 to the appearance of granulation tissue, day 1 to the start of epithelialisation, and day 1 to

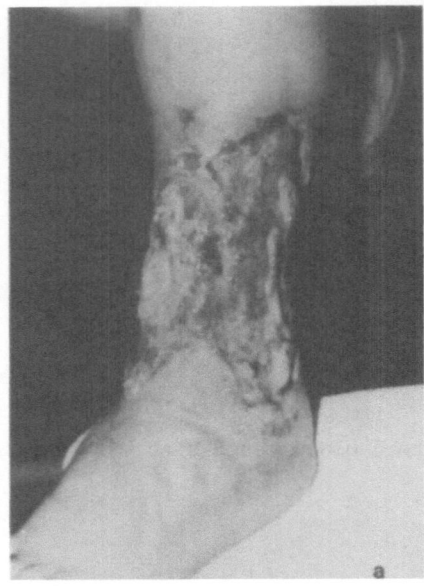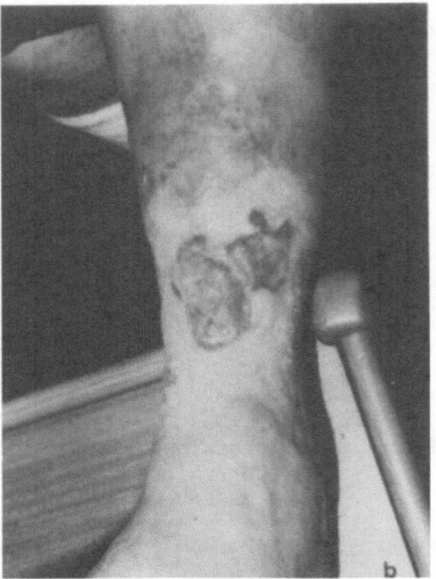

Figure 8. (a) Nonhealing venous skin ulcer in male patient (58 yrs of age) persisting for 8 months in spite of conventional treatment.

(b) Same patient as (a) 32 days later showing epithelialisation.

complete healing. In an effort to minimise observer bias the same physician assessed all patients at each stage.

The patients were divided into four groups according to ulcer size (Fig. 9, which also summarises results).

In all cases, granulation tissue appeared between the seventh and 17th day of treatment. Evidence of epithelialisation was observed between the 17th and 34th day after starting therapy (Fig. 8b; same patient as 8a). Biopsy specimens taken on day 30 showed histologically differentiated epidermis and the appearance of new capillary blood vessels (Fig. 10). The time for complete healing varied between 42 and 70 days. There were no cases of non-healing, and the age of the patient had no obvious relation to the rate of tissue repair.

Despite the general benefit of bed rest and hospital care the second untreated ulcer remained indolent in the 10 patients with bilateral ulcers. The only improvement noted was some decrease in oedema of the affected limb.

Follow-up for these 165 patients has now lasted five years. During that time only three patients have returned with small areas of breakdown of the ulcer. These have healed rapidly with further treatment. The risk of breakdown must remain if the cause of the ulcer cannot be treated.

POST-IRRADIATION CYSTITIS

The second clinical group consisted of patients suffering from post-irradiation cystitis, which can be as intractable to treatment as indolent

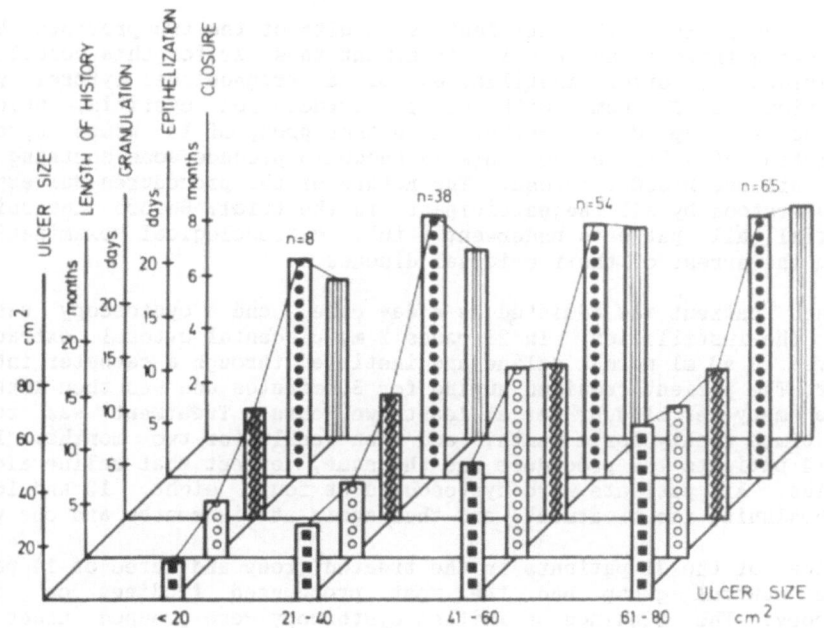

Figure 9. Relationship between the skin ulcer size and time
interval necessary to induce granulation and
epithelialisation in treated patients.

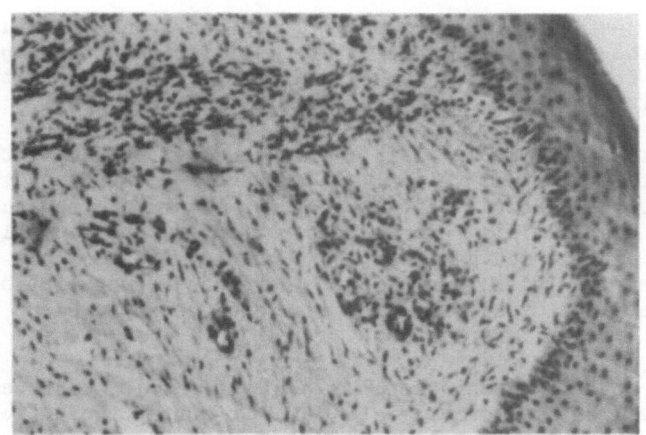

Figure 10. Skin biopsy specimen taken from the same patient as
Figure 8 on day 30 of treatment. Note differentiated
epidermis and new blood vessels (x 280).

leg ulcers. High voltage radiation therapy for carcinoma of the cervix is a
very effective therapy for this disease, but unfortunately it often gives
rise to chronic dysuria, haematuria, and frequency due to tissue damage by
the radiation. Cutaneous ureterostomy,[23] intravesicular instillation of
formalin[24] and silver nitrate[25] and, most recently, sodium pentosanpolysulphate by mouth[26] all have their advocates. In addition, since local anoxia
is responsible for the chronicity of the bladder lesion, hyperbaric oxygen
has been used as an adjunct to local treatment.[27]

On the basis of the satisfactory results of the two previous studies
and knowing there is no curative treatment thus far for this condition it
was decided to offer instillation of a trophoblast cytosol protein
preparation to 21 women with severe irradiation cystitis, which had
persisted for up to six months. A further group of 14 women agreed to
instillation of saline alone; this is known to produce some soothing effect
on the inflamed bladder mucosa. The nature of the procedures was explained
and understood by all the participants in the trial. Before admission to
the trial all patients underwent a full gynaecological examination to
confirm the arrest of their original disease.

Each patient was admitted as a day case, and a cystoscopy was done
before the instillation. In 21 cases 2 mg placental cytosol extract was
dissolved in 50 ml normal saline and instilled through a catheter into the
bladder. The patient remained supine for 30 minutes and was then instructed
not to empty her bladder for at least two hours. Treatment was repeated
three times weekly for a month, and then weekly for two months. In the
other 14 patients the procedure was the same, except that saline alone was
instilled. All patients were cystoscoped at four, eight, 12 and 16 weeks
after beginning the treatment, and then again at six months and one year.

Eight of the 21 patients in the treated group and three of 14 patients
in the control group had the most pronounced findings on initial
cystoscopy. The findings on initial cystoscopy were grouped under three
broad headings: (A) generalised redness and oedema of the bladder mucosa
in the region of the trigone and posterior bladder wall; (B) the presence,
in addition to the above, of teleangiectases, and (C) the presence of both
of the above but of a more severe nature plus pronounced incrustations of
the mucosa.

Fourteen patients in the treated group had frank haematuria at some
time during the first four weeks after instillation: eight patients from
group C; five from group B, and only one from group A. One patient required
a blood transfusion because her haemoglobin fell to 7.1 g/l.

At the first follow-up visit one month after beginning the treatment
eight patients reported relief of symptoms. Four of them had had
haematuria. On the second visit, a further 11 stated that their symptoms
had abated. The remaining two women reported symptomatic relief on their
third visit, and 15 months after the beginning of the study all 21 were
free of urinary symptoms of any kind. There was no correlation between the
type and duration of radiation treatment and the improvement produced by
the placental extract instillation.

In the control group there was no symptomatic improvement in any
patient at the first follow-up visit. At two months two patients reported
some improvement. Six months after beginning the trial six of the 14
patients were still complaining of frequency and occasional dysuria. These
six patients were originally classed group B and group C.

There is a highly significant difference in improvement between the
treated group and the control group, demonstrated by two-way analysis of
nonparametric samples by algorithm Ploshinskii.[28]

No adverse effects attributable to the placental extract were seen or
reported.

On the basis of these findings and the complete absence of any ill
effects, it would seem worth extending this placental cytosol instillation
treatment to all patients presenting with the distressing condition of
post-irradiation cystitis.[21]

DISCUSSION AND COMMENTS

The *in vivo* effects of first trimester trophoblast cytosol preparation described here indicate that some proteins of trophoblastic origin can stimulate tissue repair locally, directly inducing the whole cascade of events of the wound healing process. These effects do not appear to be species- (human, rabbit) or tissue- (cornea, skin, bladder mucosa) specific.

The pattern of events in the rabbit eye clearly shows angiogenic activity of the preparation. The complexity of the angiogenic sequence, from migration and replication of endothelial cells to budding forth of new vessels, together with the multiplication of epithelial cells and fibroblasts as part of the wound healing process, seems to favour the present belief that synergistic effects of a number of growth factors are required to effect tissue repair. The effect of our cytosol preparation, as described here, lends support to this hypothesis.

We are all aware that the use of biological material raises serious issues. Its purity, specificity and lack of standardisation are causes for concern. Consideration of such factors have persuaded some physicians that the risks attached to the use of biological material may out-weigh the benefits. However, while the risks may be the subject of informed speculation their extent and gravity are difficult to estimate, while as we have seen here the benefits can be great.

Many biological materials are in general use. Despite long experience with some of them, new knowledge comes to light from time to time giving rise to anxiety and a fresh impetus to replace them with laboratory-synthesised and standardised products. However, nothing so far produced has been sufficiently satisfactory to replace, for example, whole blood when blood is needed, and this precept seems to us to be the cornerstone of the exercise.

On the other hand, well-tested synthetic drugs have yielded some tragic surprises years after they have been in regular use and considered "safe". Examples range from beta-adrenergic blockers to non-steroidal anti-inflammatory drugs. Nevertheless, a search to find the means of analysing, purifying and eventually synthesising the beneficial factors in placental extract seems to us a matter of some importance, despite the fact that when it comes to setting up clinical trials research physicians are likely to meet a major obstacle head on. The total number of patients who might benefit from the use of these factors is unknown, and which drug manufacturer will wish to be involved in arduous and expensive research to develop a product for which the scale of use – and hence sales – cannot even be guessed at? A perfect example of what the FDA designates as an "Orphan Drug" is thus created.

This does not change our opinion that there is a good case for using placental extract in certain cases. We do not so far have a bladder instillation to mitigate the misery of irradiated patients, who are cured of their cancers, but much more ill afterwards than they ever were before being diagnosed. And we certainly need a better alternative than amputation for unsuccessful ulcer treatment.

Desperate situations require desperate measures. The Declaration of Helsinki (1975) states: "...the doctor must be free to use a new therapeutic measure if in his judgement it offers hope of saving life, re-establishing health or alleviating suffering."

Some time in the future it will be gratifying to know exactly what is the molecular structure and be able to synthesise the factor(s) that induces granulation tissue to bud and cover an enormous, leaking, denuded area of leg. In the meantime, a 76-year old patient who lives alone and can hardly cross the street from pain and incapacity does not want to have to wait until that Nobel day has dawned.

REFERENCES

1. Gruss, J.S. and Jirsch, D.W. (1978) Human amniotic membrane: a versatile wound dressing. *Can. Med. Assoc. J.* 118, 1237-1246.
2. Bose, B. (1979) Burn wound dressing with human amniotic membrane. *Ann. R. Coll. Surg. Engl.* 61, 444-447.
3. Bennett, J.P., Matthews, R. and Faulk, W.P. (1980) Treatment of chronic ulceration of the legs with human amnion. *Lancet* i, 1153-1155.
4. Faulk, W.P., Stevens, P.J., Burgos, H., Matthews, R., Bennett, J.P. and Hsi, B-L. (1980) Human amnion as an adjunct in wound healing. *Lancet* i, 1156-1157.
5. Matthews, R.N., Faulk, W.P. and Bennett, J.P. (1982) A review of the role of amniotic membranes in surgical practice. *Obstet. Gynecol. Ann.* 11, 31-57.
6. Frolik, C.A., Dart, L.L., Meyers, C.A., Smith, D.M. and Sporn, M.B. (1983) Purification and initial characterization of type β-transforming growth factor from human placenta. *Proc. Natl. Acad. Sci. USA* 80, 3676-3680.
7. Goldstein, L.D., Reynolds, C.P. and Preze-Ford, J.R. (1978) Isolation of human NGF from placental tissue. *Neurochem. Res.* 3, 175-181.
8. Gospodarowicz, D., Cheng, J., Lui, G-M., Fujii, D.K., Baird, A. and Böhlem, P. (1985) Fibroblast growth factor in the human placenta. *Biochem. Biophys. Res. Commun.* 128, 554-562.
9. O'Keefe, E.J. and Russell, N. (1985) Keratinocyte growth-promoting activity from human placenta. *J. Cell. Physiol.* 124, 439-445.
10. Burgos, H. (1983) Angiogenic and growth factors in human amniochorion and placenta. *Eur. J. Clin. Invest.* 13, 289-296.
11. Sen-Majumdar, A., Murthy, U. and Das, M. (1986) A new trophoblast-derived growth factor from human placenta: purification and receptor identification. *Biochemistry* 25, 627-634.
12. Stromberg, K., Pigott, D.A., Ranchalis, J.E. and Twardzik, D.R. (1982) Human term placenta contains transforming growth factors. *Biochem. Biophys. Res. Commun.* 106, 354-361.
13. Control of Animal Cell Proliferation (1985) Editors: A.L. Boynton and H.L. Leffert, Academic Press, Orlando.
14. Growth Factors in Biology and Medicine (1985) Ciba Foundation Symposium 116, Pitman, London.
15. Adamson, E.D. (1983) Growth factors in development. In: The Biological Basis of Reproductive and Developmental Medicine. Editor: J.B. Warshaw, Elsevier Press, New York, pp 307-336.
16. Pessa, M.E., Bland, K.L. and Copeland, E.M. (1987) Growth factors and determinants of wound repair. *J. Surg. Res.* 42, 207-217.
17. Olerud, J.E., Gown, A.M., Bickenbach, J., Dale, B. and Odland, G.F. (1988) An assessment of human epidermal repair in elderly normal subjects using immunohistochemical methods. *J. Invest. Dermatol.* 90, 845-850.
18. Chung, J-H. and Fagerholm, P. (1987) Stromal reaction and repair after corneal alkali wound in the rabbit: a quantitative microradiographic study. *Exp. Eye Res.* 45, 227-237.
19. Burstein, N.L. (1987) Review: Growth factor effects on corneal wound healing. *J. Ocul. Pharmacol.* 3, 263-277.
20. Folkman, J. (1982) Angiogenesis: initiation and control. *J. Cell Biol.* 104, 212-218.
21. Mičić, S. and Genbačev, O. (1988) Post-irradiation cystitis improved by instillation of early placental extract in saline. *Eur. Urol.* 14, 291-293.

22. Lesić, J., Dekleva, N. and Genbačev, O. (1985) Effect of placental extract-supplemented cream on epithelialisation of venous ulcers of lower leg. *Period. Biol.* **87 (2)**, 254-255.
23. Pomer, S., Karcher, G. and Simon, W. (1983) Cutaneous ureterostomy as last resort treatment of intractable haemorrhagic cystitis following radiation. *Br. J. Urol.* **55**, 392-394.
24. Firlitt, C.F. (1973) Intractable haemorrhagic cystitis secondary to extensive carcinomatosis: management with formalin solution. *J. Urol.* **110**, 57-58.
25. Kumar, A.M.P., Wrenn, E.L., Jayalakshmamma, B., Conrad, L., Quinn, P. and Cox, C. (1976) Silver nitrate irrigation to control bladder haemorrhage in children receiving cancer therapy. *J. Urol.* **116**, 85-87.
26. Parsons, C.L. (1986) Successful management of radiation cystitis with sodium pentosanpolysulphate. *J. Urol.* **136**, 813-814.
27. Weiss, J.P., Boland, F.P., Mori, H., Gallagher, M., Brereton, H., Preate, D.L. and Neville, E. (1985) Treatment of radiation-induced cystitis with hyperbaric oxygen. *J. Urol.* **134**, 352-354.
28. Ploshinskii, N.A. (1980) Biometrija. Izdatelstvo Moskovskogo Univerziteta, Moscow.

Peter Beaconsfield called the placenta "The Largest Human Biopsy"[1] and "A Neglected Experimental Animal".[2] Both descriptions are accurate. It is a readily available source of normal living human tissue (trophoblast, connective, vascular) as well as a source of proteins and peptides associated with the trophoblast - nucleic acids, lectins and collagens - to mention but a few.

As an "experimental animal" it can be maintained alive and entire at full term, and as explants or cells at any other stage under *in vitro* conditions for varying but limited periods of time.

The need for *in vitro* techniques was emphasised more than a hundred years ago by the famous French physiologist Claude Bernard, when he wrote:

" ... physiological occurrences must, as far as possible, be isolated outside the organism by means of experimental procedures. This isolation can then allow us to see and understand better the deepest associations of the phenomena, so that their vital role may be followed better in the organism."

(Leçons de physiologie experimentales, Baillière 1886)

How to use placenta as a source or an experimental animal depends entirely on the purpose of the study. There are two views concerning the study of cells and tissues. The first is that the final goal of the research is to acquire new knowledge that will result in a better understanding of what goes on *in vivo*, leading perhaps to new diagnostic methods or new treatments of particular diseases. The second embraces the alternative philosophy of studying physiological phenomena simply because they are interesting and amenable to investigation, in the hope that, eventually, some relationship to the intact organism will emerge.

As most of the contributors to this book are directly or indirectly involved with clinical medicine, they mostly fall into the first group. Thus, the relevance of the results obtained *in vitro* becomes very important for the *in vivo* situation. As all *in vitro* experiments are unphysiological in varying degrees, it is essential to establish criteria to examine their validity. For this reason, the selection and standardisation of experimental models and agreement about criteria for tissue viability are of utmost importance. These criteria fall into two major groups embracing parameters

[1] Placenta - the largest human biopsy (1982), eds. P. Beaconsfield and G. Birdwood, Pergamon Press.
[2] Placenta - a neglected experimental animal (1979), eds. P. Beaconsfield and C. Villee. Pergamon Press.

that reflect general cellular metabolism or those of the specific functions of the particular tissue or cell type.

To establish criteria for the first group and to save time, effort, and money we must define the ramic points in cellular metabolism that control and reflect the dynamic picture of cellular metabolism. Ideally, the parameters selected for such study should be a part of a routine test procedure, easy to reproduce and quick to perform. The second is much more difficult because it depends on the particular function and characteristics of the tissue.

In vitro models offer a variety of possibilities for study and each has its advantages and disadvantages. Bearing in mind that the purpose of these models is to mimic as closely as possible *in vivo* behaviour, it is important to analyse in detail the specific cellular characteristics to be investigated. All *in vitro* models provide the means of studying protein synthesis and its regulation by reducing the number of interfering factors which may be operative *in vivo*. Short-term experiments (minutes, hours) are less open to the criticism of being unphysiological. On the other hand, long-term *in vitro* experiments, in which tissue is maintained in the absence of homeostatic control for days, weeks or even months, are likely to lead to loss of cell-specific response and, consequently, to erroneous conclusions, particularly if correlation with animal or human *in vivo* data is unavailable.

Cellular synthetic and secretory activities are under the control of various mechanisms, which may be neural or endocrine, paracrine or autocrine in action. Up to the present paracrine and autocrine regulation have been almost completely ignored or little understood. By studying trophoblast, endometrium, and fetal membranes *in vitro* we can observe the phenomena of their interactions which thus far are impossible to study by any clinical techniques *in vivo*, even in experimental animals. Being readily available as the consequence of a normal physiological event and unaffected by pathological alterations as is the case with nearly all biopsy specimens, placental preparations could act as a model for the study of paracrine and autocrine regulation and indicate how the information so obtained could be applied *in vivo*.

Some important clinical problems, such as failed implantation that leads to loss of early pregnancy or unsuccessful IVF, or premature labour might be resolved by such studies, which may also provide insight into the mechanism of "hyper-implantation" and uncontrolled trophoblast invasion leading to molar pregnancies and choriocarcinoma.

Cellular secretory activity is regulated *in vivo* by a complex interplay of different factors which control release of stored or newly synthesised products. *In vitro* experiments can be used to study the direct effect of one or more factors on the release of a particular protein by measuring its concentration in the medium. When organ or tissue culture or perfusion are used nonspecific discharge from damaged cells or contamination with blood often increases the total amount of that protein in the medium. This false figure can be reduced by preincubation or equilibration of the system before the experimental procedure per se.

The release of a product can be monitored by frequent sampling of the perfusate or the incubation medium. Total replacement of the medium might lead to "shock" resulting from tissue exposure to the fresh medium, creating a sharp rise in tissue-medium gradient. Less precipitate changes (replacement of 10% of the medium at each sampling) might maintain the situation closer to the physiological state. Morphological evaluation of tissue maintained *in vitro* is important in monitoring cell interactions.

Cell polarity and ultrastructural characteristics may help to allocate a particular function to a specific cellular compartment. This approach is especially useful when organ and tissue cultures are used.

The placenta is not only an experimental model, but is also a source of biologically active products of human origin. Under normal circumstances it is a mere by-product of the newborn baby and is discarded along with the fetal membranes, umbilical cord and retroplacental blood. All this amazing harvest of normal human products is delivered into the obstetricians' hands and discarded by them to fertilise the roses. Such profligacy with nature's spontaneous gift repeated with every live normal birth would arouse passionate emotions if the placenta was better understood by more scientists.

The trophoblast still alive at delivery contains human proteins with different biological functions within its cells. Retroplacental blood is a veritable storehouse of various proteins, in particular growth factors. Trophoblast cells contain cellular synthetic machinery that might be useful in genetic manipulation. The cytosol fraction is a generous source of ribonucleic acids - different mRNAs. Its cellular membranes have multiple binding sites with differing degrees of ligand specificity. The architecture of villous structure is built up on elements of connective tissue and intercellular matrix that could be used for tissue remodelling or as a supporting matrix in plastic surgery, particularly in the treatment of burns.

The vessels of the umbilical cord and placental vessels have been used as models for training in microsurgery, and they can also be used in grafting and transplantation. The fetal membranes are the source of many biologically active compounds and attention has been drawn in this volume to their use for wound protection and healing.

In conclusion, the human placenta is a source of new information and specific biological material, and, if adequately maintained, a good experimental animal. Ideas are not lacking. Placentas are readily available without any of the ethical constraints operative in the use of other human tissues. So what are we waiting for? If it is true that placental function is still ill understood we hope the participants in our workshop and the readers of this book will want to experiment and acquire the necessary knowledge to exploit the largest human biopsy and not just consign it to the incinerator.

Olga Genbačev
Belgrade

D. R. Abramovich,
Department of Obstetrics & Gynaecology,
University of Aberdeen,
Maternity Hospital,
Cornhill Road,
Aberdeen, AB9 2ZD,
Great Britain.

J.D. Aplin,
Departments of Obstetrics & Gynaecology,
    Biochemistry & Molecular Biology,
University of Manchester,
St. Mary's Hospital,
Whitworth Park,
Manchester, M13 OJH,
England.

Rebecca Beaconsfield,
SCIP Research Unit, University of London,
Office: 23 Ennismore Avenue,
London, W4 1SE,
England.

N. A. Bersinger,
Department of Obstetrics & Gynaecology,
Division of Endocrinology,
University of Zürich,
CH-8091, Zürich,
Frauenklinkstrasse 10,
Switzerland.

H. Burgos,
Blond McIndoe Centre for Medical
    Research,
Queen Victoria Hospital,
East Grinstead,
Sussex, RH19 3DZ,
England.

Bojana Čemerikić,
Institute of Endocrinology, Immunology
    and Nutrition,
INEP,
Banatska 31b,
11080 Zemun,
Yugoslavia.

Margita Čuperlović,
Institute of Endocrinology, Immunology
    and Nutrition,
INEP,
Banatska 31b,
11080 Zemun,
Yugoslavia.

C.G. Dacke,
Department of Physiology,
University of Aberdeen,
Marischal College,
Aberdeen, AB9 1AS.
Great Britain.

P. A. di Sant'Agnese,
Department of Pathology,
University of Rochester Medical Center,
Rochester, N.Y. 14642,
USA.

R. Duft,
Department of Obstetrics & Gynaecology,
University of Berne,
CH-3012 Berne,
Schanzeneckstrasse 1,
Switzerland.

Olga Genbačev,
Institute of Endocrinology, Immunology
    and Nutrition,
INEP,
Banatska 31b,
11080 Zemun,
Yugoslavia.

A. Golander,
Departments of Pediatrics & Physiology,
Duke University,
Durham, N.C. 27710,
USA.

A. Grundis,
Department of Obstetrics & Gynecology,
Duke University,
Durham, N.C. 27710,
USA.

S. Handwerger,
Departments of Pediatrics & Physiology,
Duke University,
Durham, N.C. 27710,
USA.

I. Harman,
Departments of Pediatrics & Physiology,
Duke University,
Durham, N.C. 27710,
USA.

Karen Henderson,
Department of Obstetrics & Gynaecology,
University of Aberdeen,
Maternity Hospital,
Cornhill Road,
Aberdeen, AB9 2ZD,
Great Britain.

Miroslava Janković,
Institute of Endocrinology, Immunology
    and Nutrition,
INEP,
Banatska 31b,
11080 Zemun,
Yugoslavia.

Carolyn J. P. Jones,
Department of Pathology,
University of Manchester,
St. Mary's Hospital,
Whitworth Park,
Manchester, M13 OJH,
England.

V. Jorgensen,
Departments of Pediatrics & Physiology,
Duke University,
Durham, N.C. 27710,
USA.

A. Klopper,
Department of Obstetrics & Gynaecology,
University of Aberdeen,
Maternity Hospital,
Cornhill Road,
Aberdeen, AB9 2ZD,
Great Britain.

Jasna Lesić,
Hospital "Dr. Mladen Stojanovic",
Vinogradska 29,
Zagreb 41000,
Yugoslavia.

Dragica Ljuština,
Clinic of Ophthalmology,
Dimitrija Ducovica 161,
Belgrade 11000,
Yugoslavia.

G. Luke,
Department of Obstetrics & Gynaecology,
University of Aberdeen,
Maternity Hospital,
Cornhill Road,
Aberdeen, AB9 2ZD,
Great Britain.

A. Malek,
Department of Obstetrics & Gynaecology,
University of Berne,
CH-3012 Berne,
Schanzeneckstrasse 1,
Switzerland.

S. Mičić,
Urological Clinic,
Medical Faculty of Belgrade,
Gen. Zdanova 51,
Belgrade 11000,
Yugoslavia.

R. K. Miller,
Department of Obstetrics & Gynecology,
University of Rochester Medical Center,
601 Elmwood Avenue,
Rochester, N.Y. 14642,
USA.

G.H. Mulder,
Department of Obstetrics & Gynaecology,
Free University Hospital,
Amsterdam,
The Netherlands.

K.R. Page,
Department of Physiology,
University of Aberdeen,
Marischal College,
Aberdeen, AB9 1AS,
Great Britain.

Nada Papić,
Institute of Obstetrics & Gynaecology,
Rifata Burdzevica 31,
Belgrade 11000,
Yugoslavia.

R. Perez D'Gregorio,
National Poison Control Center,
Maternidad "Concepcion Palacios"
Unidad de Endocrinologia della
    Reproduccion,
Av. San Martin,
Caracas,
Venezuela.

R. Richards,
Departments of Pediatrics & Physiology,
Duke University,
Durham, N.C. 27710,
USA.

Risa A. Saltzman,
Department of Obstetrics & Gynecology,
University of Rochester Medical Center,
601 Elmwood Avenue,
Rochester, N.Y. 14642,
USA.

H. Schneider,
Department of Obstetrics & Gynaecology,
University of Berne,
CH-3012 Berne,
Schanzeneckstrasse 1,
Switzerland.

Y. Shah,
Department of Obstetrics & Gynecology,
University of Rochester Medical Center,
601 Elmwood Avenue,
Rochester, N.Y. 14642,
USA.

R. Sutherland,
Cancer Centre,
University of Rochester Medical Center,
Rochester, N.Y. 14642,
USA.

K. Thrailkill,
Departments of Pediatrics & Physiology,
Duke University,
Durham, N.C. 27710,
USA.

Mirjana Vučković,
Institute of Endocrinology, Immunology
    and Nutrition,
INEP,
Banatska 31b,
11080 Zemun,
Yugoslavia.

P.J. Weir
Department of Reproductive Toxicology,
Smith, Kline and French Laboratories,
PO Box 1539,
King of Prussia, Pa. 19406,
USA.

Tacey E. White,
Department of Obstetrics & Gynecology,
University of Rochester Medical Center,
601 Elmwood Avenue,
Rochester, N.Y. 14642,
USA.

Perfusion, placental, 15–78
Permeability
  amnio-chorion, effects of
      decidual prolactin on,
      103–114
  of placental membrane, studies,
      46–47
pH measurements, placental function
      during perfusion assessed
      via, 30
Phosphoinositide hydrolysis, decidual
      prolactin regulation involving,
      134
Phospholipase A2, decidual prolactin
      regulation involving, 134
Phosphorus (inorganic) measurements,
      placental function during
      perfusion assessed via, 30
Plasma protein A (pregnancy-
      associated)
  release by perfused placental
      lobules, 15–24
  synthesis by perfused placental
      lobules, 51–61 *passim*
Plasmalemma, protein passage via, 67,
      68
Post-translational modification of
      prolactin, 114
Pregnancy proteins
  categories, 51
  release from trophoblast, 63–74
    protein biosynthesis affecting,
      72–73
Pregnancy-associated proteins
  examples, 51
  release
    by perfused placental lobules,
      15–24, 64–74 *passim*
    by trophoblast, 63–74
  synthesis by perfused placental
      lobules, 51–61
Pregnancy-specific proteins
  examples, 51
  release, by trophoblast, 63–74
  synthesis by perfused placental
      lobules, 51–61
Progesterone
  decidual prolactin regulation by,
      129–130
  hCG regulation by, 93
  production by spheroid of JAr
      cells, 87, 89
  release by perfused placental
      lobules, 15, 17, 18, 20
Prolactin
  decidual, effects on amnion-chorion
      water permeability, 103–114
  general functions, 104
  hCG regulation by, 93
  pituitary and amniotic fluid,
      different activities, 110, 114

Prolactin (continued)
  production (secretion/release/
      levels), 129–135, 138
    during placental lobule
      perfusion, 15, 17, 18,
      20, 52
    factors regulating, 129–135,
      138
    inhibition, 133
    unperfused tissue, 52
Prolactin-inhibitory factor,
      decidual, 133, 135
Prolactin-releasing factor,
      decidual, 131, 135
Proliferative phase endo-
      metrium, 116
Protein(s), placental, *see
      also entries under
      Pregnancy and
      specific proteins*
  discharge, 67–69
    definition, 78
  dual perfusion for the
      study of, 39–48
  prolactin synthesis and
      release regulated
      by, 130–131
  release, 78
    definition, 78
    effects of protein biosyn-
      thesis on, 72–73, 74
    by perfused placental
      lobules, 15–24, 64–74
      passim
    from trophoblast, 64–74
  synthesis
    definition, 78
    inhibitors/uncouplers of,
      placental protein pro-
      duction during perfusion
      in presence of, 53–54, 61
    by perfused placental lobules,
      51–61
Protein kinase C, decidual
      prolactin regulation
      involving, 134
Proteoglycan distribution in
      endometrial stroma, 124
Puromycin effects
  on protein release, in tropho-
      blast explant cultures, 73
  on protein synthesis, during
      perfusion, 54, 55

Radioimmunoassay of proteins from
      pre/post-perfused tissue
      extracts, 52
Red blood cells, perfusion
      solutions containing, 28
Relaxin, decidual prolactin
      regulation by, 133

RNA splicing patterns,
    fibronectin, 124-125

Salt solutions used in perfusion,
    28
Schwangerschaftsprotein 1
  de novo synthesis by perfused
    placental lobules, 51-61
    passim
  release, 34-35, 64-74 *passim*
    by perfused placental lobules,
    15-24, 64-74 *passim*
Second messengers in cytotrophoblast,
    24
Secretory granules in intracellular
    protein transport, 68, 69
Secretory phase endometrium, 116-119,
    124
Shape of spheroids of JAr cells, 84,
    85
Size of spheroids of JAr cells, 84, 86
Soluble mammalian lectins, 145,
    146-147
Somatomedin-C (IGF-I), decidual
    prolactin regulation by,
    131-133, 135
Spheroidal culture, 81
  trophoblast in, 83-91
Stroma, endometrial
  extracellular matrix, hormone-
    dependent changes in, 115,
    116-119, 122-124
  glycosaminoglycan and proteoglycan
    distribution in, 124
Stromal cells, endometrial, breakdown
    of fibrillar matrix involving,
    124
Stromal oedema, in assessment of
    placental function during
    perfusion, 31, 32
Superfusion of fetal membranes, 64-74
    passim
Survival, *see* Viability
Syncytiotrophoblast changes, placental
    function during perfusion
    determined from, 31, 32

Thyrotrophin-releasing factor in
    placenta, 93
Tissue
  non-perfused, metabolites, studies
    of, 39-40, 41-42
  organisation, placental lectin
    involvement in, 151
  perfused
    de novo synthesised proteins in,
      measurements, 55-61
    viability, criticisms aimed at, 77
  repair, *see* Wound healing
Toxicity screening with dually
    perfused placentas, 34-35

Transport studies during dual
    placental perfusion, 31-32
Treatment with placental tissue,
    155, 161-170
  risks, 169
Trophoblast
  angiogenic and growth factor
    activity, 156, 157
  explant culture, *see*
    Explant culture
  migrating, fibronectin as an
    anchorage molecule for,
    126
  protein synthesis, 51-61
    protein release in maternal
      perfusate and,
      relationship between,
      16-24
  signals, *in vitro* models for
    reading and manipulating,
    63-74
  spheroidal culture, 83-91
  unstirred layer adjacent to,
    significance, 16
  wound healing/tissue repair
    properties, 161-170

Ulceration, treatment of
  amniotic epithelium in, 155
  trophoblast cytosol preparation
    in, 165-168
Ultrastructure
  placental function during
    perfusion determined from
    examination of, 30-31
  of spheroids of JAr cells, 86-87
Unstirred layer/volume adjacent to
    trophoblast, significance,
    16, 21

Varicose ulcers, amniotic epithe-
    lium in treatment of, 155
Vascularisation (neo-), trophoblast
    cytosol preparation-induced,
    163, 164
Vasculature, fetal, placental
    function during perfusion
    determined from, 29-30
Viability
  of perfused tissue, criticisms
    aimed at, 77
  of trophoblast explants, 94
Virus movement across placenta
    during dual perfusion, 32
Vitamin B_{12} transport during
    placental perfusion, 31-32
Water
  permeability, amnio-chorion,
    effects of decidual
    prolactin on, 103-114